THE
THYROID
FIX

THE
THYROID
FIX

The No-Nonsense Guide to **Fix Fatigue, Fogginess,** and **Fat** That Won't Budge

---

DR. AMIE HORNAMAN

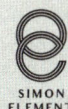

SIMON
ELEMENT

*New York Amsterdam/Antwerp London
Toronto Sydney/Melbourne New Delhi*

SIMON
ELEMENT

An Imprint of Simon & Schuster, LLC
1230 Avenue of the Americas
New York, NY 10020

This publication contains the opinions and ideas of its author. It is intended to provide helpful and informative material on the subjects addressed in the publication. It is sold with the understanding that the author and publisher are not engaged in rendering medical, health, or any other kind of personal professional services in the book. The reader should consult his or her medical, health or other competent professional before adopting any of the suggestions in this book or drawing inferences from it.

The author and publisher specifically disclaim all responsibility for any liability, loss or risk, personal or otherwise, which is incurred as a consequence, directly or indirectly, of the use and application of any of the contents of this book.

Simon & Schuster strongly believes in freedom of expression and stands against censorship in all its forms. For more information, visit BooksBelong.com.

For information about special discounts for bulk purchases, please contact Simon & Schuster Special Sales at 1-866-506-1949 or business@simonandschuster.com.

The Simon & Schuster Speakers Bureau can bring authors to your live event. For more information or to book an event, contact the Simon & Schuster Speakers Bureau at 1-866-248-3049 or visit our website at www.simonspeakers.com.

Interior design by Silverglass

Manufactured in the United States of America

1 3 5 7 9 10 8 6 4 2

The Library of Congress Cataloging-in-Publication Data has been applied for.

ISBN 978-1-6682-2542-4
ISBN 978-1-6682-2544-8 (ebook)

Scan here to get book recommendations, exclusive offers, and more delivered to your inbox.

Most people skip reading the dedication, but I need
you to pause here, because this one is about *you*.

To every woman who has sat in her car and cried after another
doctor said, "You're fine." To every patient who has trusted
me with her story and shown me just how heavy this journey
can be. To every woman still searching for answers even after
being dismissed as "normal." To every woman who knows
something is wrong in her body but can't get anyone to listen.
This book is dedicated to you and your strength. It is my
promise that you are not forgotten, and you are not alone.

Contents

THE
THYROID
FIX

The Silent Epidemic

I'm calling it what it is: a silent epidemic. You won't hear about it on the news, there are no flashy headlines, but thyroid dysfunction is everywhere. It's hitting millions of people, mostly women, and leaving them stuck in bodies that don't feel like their own.

According to the American Thyroid Association, roughly one in eight Americans has some form of thyroid dysfunction, and nearly 5 percent of Americans over the age of twelve have hypothyroidism, a condition in which the thyroid gland fails to produce enough thyroid hormone. This astonishing statistic amounts to over 30 million people, just slightly less than the number of Americans who have high blood pressure or diabetes. Yet I believe, based on what I see in my practice, that thyroid dysfunction is still largely underdiagnosed, undertested, and undertreated. Recent research suggests that the true rate of hypothyroidism is closer to 10 to 12 percent of the US population and climbing.[1] This doesn't even take into account the many subclinical cases where thyroid dysfunction is already brewing and impacting people's lives but is not severe enough to be diagnosed or flagged through testing by most providers.

Today, there are millions of people walking around with weight gain, fatigue, hair loss, brain fog, constipation, and the many other life-altering symptoms of hypothyroidism—all while being told that their lab tests are "normal." These people are invisible. And that's why I call this a silent epidemic. There are no national awareness campaigns, no research funding being poured into thyroid dysfunction diagnosis and treatment. There's no special ribbon that people pin to their shirts or lapels. It flies under the radar, and that may be because women are five to eight times as likely to be impacted by it as men are.[2] Even though hypothyroidism is highly treatable, when it comes to women's health in general, we are too often dismissed, our symptoms minimized, and our suffering normalized.

Thyroid dysfunction also remains underdiagnosed because providers don't run the right tests. Ask most MDs and DOs how much training they got on the thyroid in medical school, and they'll tell you, "We learned to test for TSH." And that's it. They were taught to order a blood test for thyroid-stimulating hormone (TSH), which isn't even a thyroid hormone, by the way; it's a brain hormone, produced by the pituitary gland in the brain. It is the messenger that pokes your thyroid and says, "Hey, buddy, time to wake up and get to work." But the presence or absence of TSH alone does not tell us whether your thyroid is working well, and it certainly doesn't provide enough information to tell us why you put on ten pounds in a month or why you are losing your hair in clumps. Your TSH level is only an indicator of how well your pituitary gland is nudging your thyroid—but your thyroid could be falling asleep at the wheel, and your pituitary might not be yelling loud enough, even if your TSH level is "normal." Too often doctors will glance at your TSH test results, stamp you "fine," and send you out the door. But if they test only for TSH, you're not getting the full picture. Period.

If you're a woman in perimenopause or menopause, getting a diagnosis can be even trickier. That's when the symptoms caused by natural hormonal changes and the symptoms of thyroid dysfunction start overlapping like a Venn diagram from Hell. I call this scenario *thyropause*, and no, it's not in the medical textbooks, but it should be. Thyropause is when your thyroid gland—please pardon my expression—shits the bed after the age of forty due to your fluctuating hormones. These fluctuations create enough stress on the body to flip the thyroid dysfunction switch to the "on" position. It's incredibly common, and it's why so many women who come to me say, "You know, it was after I turned forty that things started falling apart." Disentangling these symptoms and identifying their root causes take awareness and expertise, and sadly, many doctors today aren't up for the challenge. They focus on one or two test results and miss the bigger picture.

This is how we've ended up with a silent epidemic. It's silent because providers don't run the right labs; silent because women's symptoms are too often dismissed as aging or menopause; silent because when we complain of exhaustion, weight gain, or depression, we're told to eat less and move more or handed a prescription for antidepressants. Silent because women are conditioned not to question authority, so we walk away sheepishly, second-guessing ourselves instead of demanding answers.

Meanwhile, your body is screaming. It's rebelling. And no one is listening. But I am. And I'll keep screaming about it until people finally wake up.

Here's the truth: Your body was not built to be fat, foggy, and fatigued. We were built to be vibrant. We were built to thrive. We should not be gaining weight just by looking sideways at a brownie. We should not be crashing at 2:00 p.m. like we need a nap just to survive the day. We should not be collecting clumps of hair in the shower and wondering if we could knit a small sweater out of them.

We deserve better. You can feel better and *be* better. In this book, I'm going to show you how.

Been There, Suffered That

Before I became "The Thyroid Fixer," I was an overweight kid who was teased, bullied, and painfully aware that I didn't look like the other girls. Every day before school, I was in the living room sweating through Jane Fonda or *Buns of Steel* VHS tapes. I wasn't working out because I loved movement; I was desperately trying to change my body before my age even hit double digits.

By the time I turned sixteen and could finally join a gym, I was hooked on the idea of having control over how I looked. I dived into step classes and learned to use every Nautilus machine. That turned into teaching step aerobics, then spin classes, and eventually becoming a certified personal trainer. Fitness became my identity, but deep down, it was still rooted in a desire not to be the girl everyone made fun of.

In my early twenties, I dated a bodybuilder, which opened up an entirely new world of fitness. I got a taste of the competition lifestyle and began training and living like a figure athlete. My body transformed, and I learned what was possible if I worked hard and followed the plan. My first event was the EAS Body for Life Challenge, and I went on to compete in additional figure competitions. I worked with a trainer who was the go-to coach for fitness models at the time, and he knew exactly how to get results.

But let me be very clear: I fought for every ounce of muscle I gained and every pound of fat I lost. No matter how hard I trained, my body's default was storing fat, especially around my belly. My solution was to live in a constant state of restriction. I ate lean protein and green vegetables on repeat. I meal prepped obsessively on Sundays. I skipped social events. I didn't drink. I took Tupperware with my own food to restaurants. I followed every healthy eating and weight loss rule to the letter, because slipping up felt like going backward.

Then, after I had been competing and modeling for about six years, for the first time ever, the scale started going up . . . first five pounds, then ten. And I wasn't doing anything differently. In fact, I was being stricter than usual. When I messaged my coach, he accused me of cheating on my diet. That hit hard. I wasn't cheating. I was doing everything exactly as prescribed, and more.

The shame I thought I'd buried came rushing back. I found myself wearing oversized sweatshirts to the gym again to hide my body. I was convinced that everyone was staring at me, judging me. I started wondering if I should add more cardio, cut my calories even further, or start skipping meals. Something didn't make sense to me, though. My habits hadn't changed, yet my body had turned against me. I felt like I was failing at something I had worked so hard to master.

I didn't know where to turn. My sister, who's a doctor, was my first call. She did blood work and went through every possibility she could think of, but when my labs came back, she said, "Amie, everything is normal."

I kept pushing for answers and asking questions, but there was no obvious reason for my weight gain. Finally, my sister referred me to a metabolic disease specialist. I thought I'd hit the jackpot. The man had "metabolism" in his title, after all. He would understand what I was going through.

I prepped for that appointment as though it were a job interview. I brought along food logs, workout notes, lab results, and symptom journals. I explained everything from how hard I was working out to how dramatically my body was changing without any apparent cause. The doctor listened briefly, glanced at my labs, and then told me that everything was "within normal range." That word, *normal*, became a trigger. Nothing about my body felt normal. He pointed to where I was on a body mass index (BMI) chart and said that I was "fine." And then came the line I would hear more than once: "Just eat less and exercise more."

I walked out of that office, sat in my car, put my head on the steering wheel, and sobbed. At that point, I would have welcomed *any* diagnosis— something, anything, to name what was happening to me. Even a scary one would've been better than "You're fine." Because I wasn't fine, and as I'd tried to tell anyone who would listen, it was more than just rapid, inexplicable weight gain. My hair was thinning. My energy had tanked, and I was living on Monster energy drinks. I was faking it through training sessions, hiding under baggy clothes and behind a forced smile. I stopped weighing myself when I hit twenty-five pounds of unexplained weight gain. I felt like a stranger in my own body. But it wasn't just about how I looked; it was about losing control over my health, body, and identity.

I ultimately saw six doctors over the next year. Each one dismissed me. Each one told me I was fine—until finally, doctor number seven did something different. She touched my throat during a routine exam and paused. "You've got a nodule on your thyroid," she said. "We'll confirm it with an ultrasound, but I believe you have hypothyroidism."

For the first time, I felt as though someone was seeing me. And when the ultrasound confirmed her diagnosis, I was relieved. I finally had a name for what was happening: hypothyroidism, specifically Hashimoto's thyroiditis, an autoimmune disease in which your body makes antibodies that attack the cells in your thyroid gland. As a result, you can't produce enough thyroid hormone for your body's needs, which explained everything I had been experiencing, from the sudden weight gain to the fatigue.

The doctor wrote me a prescription for levothyroxine, the most common thyroid medication, and said it would help. I thought, "This is it. I'm going to feel like myself again." But I didn't. Months passed, and nothing changed. Not my weight or my energy. Not my hair or my mood. I was still dragging. So I turned to the only other doctor I had access to, the one that is always available for questions: Dr. Google.

I researched everything I could about hypothyroidism. That was when I discovered what my doctor had never told me: Levothyroxine is a synthetic version of T4, one of the four thyroid hormones produced by your thyroid, but it is *inactive*. In fact, T4 is the stored form of T3, the *active* thyroid hormone that influences almost every biochemical process in your body. We have to convert T4 into T3 for it to be useful, and if our bodies aren't converting well? We're out of luck. I discovered that some doctors prescribe T4 and T3 together or even T3 alone. That made sense to me. Why not give the body what it needs? I printed out studies, highlighted paragraphs, and took them to my doctor like a student presenting a thesis.

She didn't even look at the papers. "No," she said. "That's not the standard of care."

I tried to reason with her. "I'm not asking you to go rogue," I told her. "I just want to try something that might help me."

She shook her head. A firm no. And that was when I knew I was on my own. Again. But this time, I had a clear direction. The questions I could now ask were the ones that would lead me to answers, not just for myself but for thousands of others like me who were tired of being dismissed, misdiagnosed, and only minimally treated. I pursued the world of functional and integrative medicine because I needed to understand the options for *anything* that wasn't "standard of care." At last I found a functional medicine doctor named Dr. Len Brancewicz, who asked me the single most impactful question anyone in medicine can ask: "How do you feel?"

I knew I was finally in the right place. Dr. Len didn't just see a lab result; he saw *me* and listened to my story. He spent ninety minutes with me, not the twelve to fifteen minutes I'd gotten from doctors one through seven. He treated me like a whole human being and asked me about everything: my medical history, symptoms, sleep patterns, digestion, nutrition, stress, workouts, and mindset. He looked at the twenty-five-plus pounds I had gained in such a short time and said, "That's not normal"—not because it didn't fit onto a BMI chart but because it didn't fit with who I was. He acknowledged that my symptoms weren't random or imaginary. The best part was that he believed they could be fixed.

Then came the move that changed it all for me: He added T3 to my treatment plan. That tiny adjustment was what flipped the switch on how I felt.

The weight started to come off. The fog lifted. My energy came back. My hair not only stopped falling out, but new hair started growing. I could get out of bed in the morning without dragging, and when I worked out, I saw results.

There's nothing more powerful than looking in the mirror and finally recognizing yourself again. That moment, when your body starts working *with* you instead of against you, is indescribable. I wasn't just lighter on the scale; I felt as though I had finally climbed out of a body that wasn't mine and stepped back into the one that had been waiting for me.

Dr. Len didn't just give me back my health, he inspired the next chapter of my life and became my mentor. I went back to school and earned my master's and doctoral degrees in clinical nutrition and became certified in functional medicine. I knew I had to help other people the way he had helped me. Today, I have a thriving practice, the Advanced Thyroid and Hormone Clinic, that has helped thousands of women all across the country fix their thyroids and reclaim their lives.

My story isn't rare, which is why I'm sharing it with you. Because if a fit, disciplined, twentysomething-year-old doing everything "right" could be misdiagnosed and dismissed by seven doctors in a major US medical system, you better believe it is happening to millions of others. I wrote this book so that you don't have to cycle through seven doctors before someone listens to you. I wrote it so you will have the tools to decode what your body is telling you, find the right help, and finally feel like yourself again.

Above all, I want you to know that there are answers. There are real, lasting solutions. You do not have to settle for being told you are "normal" when you feel anything but. With the right treatment protocol, you can feel strong, energized, and fully alive again. It happened for me, and it can happen for you, too.

. . .

In my practice, I see women every day who've spent months, sometimes years, trying to push through. They hope that things will just get better, but eventually the symptoms pile up and they can't explain them away anymore. That's when they show up in my world, tired, frustrated, and sometimes on the verge of tears. In my experience, these women fall into two groups.

The first group is the *undiagnosed*. These are the people who know something's off. They're exhausted, gaining weight, losing hair, and battling mood swings or brain fog, but they've been told they're fine. Maybe their labs came back "normal." Maybe no one ran the right tests. They might be told that it's just aging, that their symptoms are caused by stress, or that it's "just life." But they know better. They're googling symptoms, jumping from diet to diet, and wondering why their body isn't cooperating. They feel dismissed and unheard, and they're desperate for real answers.

The second group is the *undertreated*. These are the people who've finally gotten a diagnosis, usually hypothyroidism or Hashimoto's thyroiditis, but they're still not getting the help they need. They may be on medication, maybe a T4 replacement such as Synthroid, but they don't feel any improvement. Sometimes they feel worse. They've taken their concerns to their doctor, only to be told once again that everything looks "normal" and that this is all that can be done.

This book is for the women in both camps who are tired of being dismissed as though their symptoms are all in their heads, of trying everything and still feeling as if they're falling apart.

My patient Janet is an example of someone who had been doing everything right. She'd been eating clean, working out, staying on top of life as best she could. But her energy was gone, her mind was foggy, her clothes didn't fit, and she barely recognized the person looking back at her in the mirror. She'd done enough googling to suspect hormones or thyroid, but her primary care doctor ran a few basic labs and told her she was fine. Her ob-gyn said that it was probably perimenopause and told her the same things about eating and exercise that I had heard years before and that you have probably heard, too. Meanwhile, her performance at work was slipping, her confidence was shot, and there was growing tension in her marriage. When she walked into my office, she wasn't just tired, she was terrified.

Janet is the typical undiagnosed thyroid case, walking around undiagnosed and unsupported. These people are vulnerable to all the flashy wellness marketing out there. Adrenal cleanses. Gut resets. Several-hundred-dollar programs that promise fat loss in thirty days. Undiagnosed people are desperate to find anything that makes sense, so they try it all. Eventually, many of them discover that their thyroid was the missing piece of the puzzle all along.

Then there are the undertreated folks like my patient Rebecca. Rebecca never bounced back after her first pregnancy. She received a diagnosis of hypothyroidism when her primary care doctor ran basic blood work and was prescribed levothyroxine, a standard replacement for T4. She took it faithfully, but months passed and the weight stayed and the fatigue grew. Her toddler started sleeping through the night, but she didn't. She asked her doctor questions and was handed an antidepressant; no new tests, no changes to her thyroid medication. She started searching for answers, landed in Facebook groups, and finally found people like me, who told her that the pill she was taking works for less than the tip of the iceberg of hypothyroid patients and, most important, that she wasn't crazy. Rebecca had gotten stuck in the cycle of conventional care in which everything is treated in isolation and normal labs are the end of the conversation. In reality, she needed more than her doctor was trained to give.

Janet and Rebecca were living on opposite ends of the same broken system. One of them was ignored, the other minimized. Both were dismissed. And both were suffering from a very real medical condition that robbed them of their energy, clarity, confidence, and quality of life.

The tragedy wasn't that they had thyroid dysfunction; it was that no one saw it. No one caught it early, and no one treated it effectively. If they had, everything could have been different.

∙ ∙ ∙

If your story is similar to mine or to Janet's and Rebecca's, this book is for you. It is for every woman who is tired of her symptoms being dismissed as though they're all in her head.

In my practice, every patient I see is treated as an individual and not a lab result. I give her a plan that is personalized, reviewed regularly, and adjusted based on how she *feels*. My approach is a blend of conventional and functional medicine. I'm not anti-medication. In fact, I'll be the first to say that most people with hypothyroidism need medication. I did. My patients do. A green smoothie and a stack of supplements won't replace thyroid hormones when your body isn't producing them. That's the reality. What I *am* against is a health care system that provides only Band-Aid solutions and cookie-cutter care and whose practitioners throw pills at people while ignoring how they feel. When it comes to hypothyroidism, textbook treatment protocols are insufficient for many women. Learning about the "dual treatment" approach that combines prescription T3 with T4 changed so much for me. It gave me my life back.

Healing is never one-size-fits-all. I firmly believe that the worst thing a practitioner can do is pick one modality and treat it like gospel. This book will arm you with the information and tools to find a doctor or practitioner who is willing to look at everything, adjust and adapt where necessary, and stay in the game with you. Hypothyroidism, especially in women, needs ongoing attention. One little shift in stress, our larger hormonal landscape, or our nutrient status can throw everything off. Maintaining thyroid health is often a work in progress, and it needs to be managed as such.

This book puts that philosophy into your hands. It will give you the clarity and confidence to ask better questions and advocate for better care. I am here to treat you like the intelligent, capable person you are, not a passive bystander waiting for someone else to figure it out. Because you know your body. And you deserve a provider who respects that.

I've lived and studied this, and I've helped thousands of other people walk the thyroid treatment path. I want that for you, too. This is your road map, a guide to reclaiming your health, energy, confidence, and ultimately your life. From this point forward, we're in the trenches together, battling through the weight gain, the brain fog, the fatigue—all of it.

Let's fix this together. Your journey to healing starts now.

Self-Assessment: Is It Your Thyroid?

Now that you know my story, you might be starting to suspect that the symptoms you've been experiencing and thought were random . . . probably aren't.

So it's time to look at your experience. This is your moment to be completely honest. You don't have to downplay your symptoms to keep someone in a white coat comfortable or sugarcoat your struggles because you're afraid of being labeled dramatic. This self-assessment questionnaire will help you begin to connect the dots between your symptoms and your personal history and determine whether your thyroid may be to blame. But this is only a first step. No matter your result, keep reading to learn more about thyroid health and the many options for treatment that can help you get back to feeling your best.

SELF-ASSESSMENT QUESTIONNAIRE
Answer yes or no to the following questions.

Section 1: Family History
1. Has anyone in your family been diagnosed with hypothyroidism or Hashimoto's thyroiditis?

2. Does anyone in your immediate family have an autoimmune condition such as Crohn's disease, rheumatoid arthritis, or celiac disease?

3. Have you been diagnosed with an autoimmune condition yourself, for example lupus, multiple sclerosis, or type 1 diabetes?

Section 2: Symptoms
1. Have you gained weight unexpectedly in the last six months without changes in your diet or exercise?

2. Are you experiencing weight loss resistance, where weight will not come off no matter what you do?

3. Are you experiencing hair loss or hair thinning?

4. Do you feel extreme fatigue during the day, even after a full night's sleep?

5. Are you dealing with constipation or sluggish digestion?

6. Are you experiencing anxiety or depression that does not seem connected to a specific life event or situation?

7. Do you often have brain fog, forgetfulness, or difficulty concentrating?

8. Do you struggle to recover after workouts, or does exercise drain your energy for the rest of the day?

9. Do you have joint pain, such as frozen shoulder, or stiffness without a clear cause?

10. Are you unusually cold when everyone else is comfortable?

11. Are you unusually warm when everyone else is comfortable?

12. Have you noticed a loss of hairs on the outer edge of your eyebrows?

13. Do you have dry skin, brittle nails, or dry eyes?

Section 3: Additional Indicators

1. Have you been diagnosed with hypothyroidism or Hashimoto's thyroiditis and are still experiencing symptoms, with or without treatment?

2. Do you have irregular menstrual cycles, heavy periods, or other unexplained changes in your menstrual health?

3. Have you experienced infertility or recurrent miscarriages?

4. Do you frequently feel weak or have low energy levels that interfere with your daily activities?

5. Do you have issues with blood sugar regulation, such as getting "hangry" if you don't eat every few hours or experiencing spikes and crashes?

6. Have you been diagnosed with insulin resistance despite eating a low-carbohydrate diet?

SCORING

0–3 yes answers: Knowledge is power!
You bought this book; you might as well keep reading. Your health will still benefit! Even if your score is low, you came to the right place. Thyroid issues can exist without the classic symptoms or may be in the early stages. Many of the symptoms associated with thyroid dysfunction can also result from hormone imbalances, nutrient deficiencies, or chronic stress. In the chapters ahead, you'll learn how your thyroid impacts nearly every aspect of your health and how optimizing its function can unlock more energy, weight regulation, and vitality. Even if you're not sure that thyroid dysfunction applies to you yet, the tools in this book can help you build resilience and improve your overall health.

4–7 yes answers: Your symptoms deserve attention!
Your answers suggest that your symptoms may be connected to a thyroid imbalance. It's common for people with this score

to feel frustrated; perhaps you've been told that your labs are "normal," but your body is clearly telling you that something is off. Symptoms such as fatigue, weight struggles, hair loss, and brain fog often go unnoticed or dismissed, but they are not normal and shouldn't be ignored. In the chapters ahead, you'll learn why these symptoms are so common and how they connect to thyroid health. You'll also discover steps you can take to finally feel like yourself again.

8+ yes answers: A clear sign of thyroid dysfunction!
Your score strongly suggests a thyroid issue such as hypothyroidism or Hashimoto's thyroiditis, and it's likely that you've been struggling with these symptoms for some time. Maybe you've tried diets, exercise programs, or even supplements, yet nothing seems to work. You may have even been diagnosed, but the treatment hasn't resolved your symptoms. This book will walk you through everything you need to know about your thyroid, including why conventional approaches often fail and how to optimize your thyroid function. By continuing to read, you'll discover how to take control of your health, find the right treatments, and regain the energy, focus, and vitality you deserve.

WHY YOUR SCORE MATTERS
Your score is not just a number; it's a reflection of how well your body is functioning and what it is trying to tell you. Whether your score is low, moderate, or high, your thyroid is at the core of your metabolism, energy, and overall well-being. The pages ahead will not only teach you how to understand your thyroid better but also reveal the exact steps you can take to transform your health. You'll learn how to ask for the right lab tests, interpret your results, and implement strategies for true healing.

PART I

Wake Up and Smell the Thyroid Dysfunction

Chapter 1

Listen to Your Body, That's Your Thyroid Talking

You've gone to doctor after doctor and specialist after specialist, and I bet you've heard things like "You're just getting older" and "You're perfectly normal." But you know your body, and you know when something isn't right. You *feel* it. And all you want to do is scream, "Can someone please just figure out what the hell is going on with me?"

I tell every patient who walks through my door: The problem is not you, the problem is your thyroid and the way it's being ignored. I then begin by explaining a few key facts. First, thyroid function declines with age for all of us; it's inevitable. But when multiple symptoms come on quickly, that's not just aging. That's *thyropause*. Thyropause is what happens when your thyroid goes haywire due to the hormone fluctuations that accompany perimenopause. The decline in estrogen and progesterone adversely impacts your thyroid function, triggering hypothyroidism, which all too often goes untreated until it starts causing real problems. And when your thyroid is underperforming, other systems start collapsing, too. Your blood pressure rises. Your cholesterol climbs. Your blood sugar spikes. You end up with a cascade of health issues that affect almost every organ and physiological process in your body.

Your thyroid is small but mighty. And when it's underperforming, you don't just feel "off"; you feel as though you've lost yourself completely. Let's take a closer look at this all-powerful gland to understand how exactly it is supposed to work, and how it underpins—and can undermine—so much of our well-being and health.

Thyroid 101

Your thyroid is a small butterfly-shaped gland at the base of your neck that ever so quietly runs the show. It is your body's power plant, thermostat, and control center all in one. When it's working right, you don't think about it; you enjoy life in what I call "Optimization Land," the place where your thyroid functions beautifully and all your thyroid hormone levels are exactly as nature designed. Optimization Land is a wonderful place to live in where you have abundant energy throughout the entire day, you don't gain weight just by thinking about a bowl of pasta bolognese, and you actually *want* to have sex *and* work out. Not only that, you also enjoy a clear mind, a balanced mood, good sleep, and healthy digestion. Sound amazing? That's how much power your thyroid truly has.

When all your body's systems are firing on all cylinders, it's easy to forget how many moving parts are working behind the scenes to keep it that way. The thyroid doesn't just sit there pumping out hormones—which serve as your body's chemical messengers—at random. It's part of a bigger communication system that keeps every process in your body on mission. Believe it or not, every single cell in your body has a receptor on its surface for thyroid hormone, which means that your thyroid and the four hormones it produces—T1, T2, T3, and T4—influence everything from your brain to your gut.

The thyroid doesn't operate solo. Instead, it is part of a crucial chain of command called the hypothalamic-pituitary-thyroid (HPT) axis. The hypothalamus is a region of the brain that sits right above the pituitary gland and plays a crucial role in regulating bodily functions such as heart rate and digestion, and in maintaining homeostasis. It sends signals to the pituitary, known as the "master gland," which in turn sends out hormones that direct the function of other glands, including the thyroid. I like to think of the HPT axis as a well-organized military operation.

The hypothalamus is the general that sets the mission. It sends orders to the pituitary, the commanding officer, which then gives instructions to the thyroid, the field captain, to deploy thyroid hormones where they're needed. When the chain of command is strong, the mission runs smoothly. But if communication breaks down, orders get mixed up and the whole operation starts to fall apart.

The line of communication between the pituitary and the thyroid is a chemical messenger called thyroid-stimulating hormone (TSH). TSH is what nudges the thyroid to produce T1, T2, T3, and T4. Think of the pituitary as a sensor that constantly checks whether there are enough thyroid hormones circulating in your body to keep all your systems running smoothly. When levels drop, the sensor goes off and the pituitary sends out TSH, which spurs the thyroid into action to make the hormones your body needs.

Each of the four thyroid hormones has its own mission and purpose, but together they determine how well your body performs every single day.

- **T4 (thyroxine)** is the inactive, "storage" form of T3. T4 is kind of like supplies sitting in a warehouse; it doesn't do much until your body needs it. When demand for T3 increases, T4 can be converted into T3 by the liver, kidneys, and brain. About 80 percent of what your thyroid produces is T4.
- **T3 (triiodothyronine)** is the active hormone, the one out in the field doing the work. Every cell in your body has a receptor site for T3. It enters your cells and tells them to create energy, burn fat, and regulate body temperature. It also helps regulate neuronal excitability and synaptic transmission in your brain, influencing your mood as well as your memory and concentration. Even the mitochondria (the "powerhouses" of your cells) need T3 to produce ATP, your body's energy currency. When T3 is low, everything slows down. You feel tired, foggy, bloated, and disconnected from your usual vigor and vitality.

T3 has two forms, bound and free. Bound T3 is attached to a carrier protein (usually thyroxine-binding globulin, or TBG) that prevents it from entering your cells, whereas free T3 is the unbound, biologically active, usable form of T3 that can bind to cell receptors, get inside the cells, and influence cell function. Bound T3 creates a large, stable reservoir of T3 that your body can use as needed, and in fact it makes up 99 percent of the T3 circulating in your bloodstream at any given time. But free T3 is what determines how energized and alive you feel. You can have plenty of total T3, but if most of it is tied up and unavailable, your body will still feel sluggish. While you can get a blood test that measures your total T3, I believe this test is largely irrelevant. A free T3 test, which measures the *active* form of T3, is the one that really matters.

- **T2 (3,5-diiodo-L-thyronine)** is the forgotten hero of the thyroid team. It helps increase your basal metabolic rate, improves your fat burning, and keeps your mitochondria running efficiently. T2 is what helps your body say no to fat storage and yes to energy.[1] While most doctors don't address T2, I believe it has an important role to play in thyroid health—see chapter 10.

- **T1 (monoiodothyronine)** is still being studied and may play a role in cellular signaling. However, it does not bind to the same cell receptors as T3 and T4 and does not require correction in cases of thyroid dysfunction.

All four thyroid hormones are composed of tyrosine, an amino acid, and iodine, an essential mineral. In fact, the numbers associated with T1, T2, T3, and T4 refer to how many iodine atoms each type of thyroid molecule has. It should be no surprise, then, that iodine itself plays an essential role in thyroid health—despite many myths to the contrary. I'll talk more about the importance of iodine as a nutritional supplement in chapter 9.

The Thyroid Effect

Your thyroid plays an enormous role in almost every physiological process in your body. When it's steady and strong and functioning as it should, every other system knows what to do. But when it falters, everything gets messy. That's when symptoms start piling up: fatigue, brain fog, weight gain, anxiety, hair loss, mood swings. It's not that your body is broken, it's that the field captain has gone quiet.

Here are some of the ways in which your thyroid impacts your overall health.

- Your thyroid controls your metabolism. It has the final say on whether you burn those extra ten pounds or store them forever on your hips and thighs.[2] Thyroid hormones ensure that your cells burn calories efficiently, can raise or lower your basal metabolic rate, and can even change fat cells to be metabolically active[3] so that your overall body fat percentage remains low.

- Your thyroid keeps your energy up. T3 binds directly to your mitochondria, the "powerhouses" inside your cells that convert molecules from the food you eat into units of energy in the form adenosine triphosphate (ATP). T3 can also increase the number of mitochondria in each cell.[4] The more ATP you produce, the better you feel.

- Your heart rate, heart rhythm, and blood pressure are all directly impacted by thyroid hormone. Too much T3— a condition called hyperthyroidism—can cause arrhythmias and increase your risk of stroke. Too little T3 can cause a slowing of your heart rate, constriction of your blood vessels, and increased blood pressure. But at the right level, T3 optimizes the functioning of your entire cardiovascular system.

- Digestion is highly influenced by thyroid hormones, and an underperforming thyroid slows the digestive process, leading to poor nutrient absorption, bloating, gas, and constipation. A healthy thyroid is actually what helps you poop regularly.

- Your brain relies on thyroid hormones, which play a direct role in mood as well as cognitive processes such as memory and concentration. Because these hormones are so important, the brain is one of the sites for T4 to T3 conversion. A sluggish thyroid can lead to feelings of anxiety or just feeling "meh" and sap your mental clarity.

- Your ovaries depend on thyroid hormones to keep your cycle regular and support ovulation. When your thyroid function slows, your cycle can become irregular, your fertility drops, and your risk of miscarriage goes up. It's one of the main reasons thyroid health is so tied to women's health.

- Even cholesterol is under thyroid control. When thyroid function is low, your liver doesn't get the signal to clear cholesterol from the blood. So your cholesterol goes up, not because of your diet but because your thyroid stopped giving the right instructions.

   For all these reasons, optimizing your thyroid health promises a better life, not just fewer symptoms. When your thyroid is functioning well, every other system in your body is protected.

The Conversion Conversation: How T3 Is Made from T4

As we saw above, T4 accounts for 80 percent of the hormone your thyroid gland produces, but it is inactive until it is converted into T3. I like to think of T4 and T3 as being like money in the bank: T4 is your savings account, stored and safe but not doing anything for you until you transfer it into checking; T3 is your checking account, the "money" you actually get to spend on energy, metabolism, and feeling alive.

The T4 to T3 conversion happens mostly in the liver and gut; a smaller percentage inside the thyroid gland itself; and the rest in tissues such as your muscles, brain, and kidneys. It requires the help of certain enzymes, most notably deiodinase type 1 (D1) and deiodinase type 2 (D2). Think of these enzymes as little workers that turn the raw material (T4) into the good stuff (T3) that powers your metabolism, your energy, your brain, your mood, and almost everything else. But here's the thing: The conversion process is *not* easy. I always say that it's like running ten Tough

Mudders in a row: It's hard work for your body, and a lot can go wrong along the way. If it's not happening properly, you can look "normal" on paper and still feel exhausted, heavy, and far from optimal.

The conversion process depends on several factors. You need key nutrients such as selenium, iodine, zinc, magnesium, and iron. You also need a healthy gut and liver. If your gut is inflamed or your liver is overburdened with toxins or stress, the T4 to T3 conversion will slow down.[5] Chronic stress, high cortisol, infections, inflammation, calorie restriction, and even certain medications can all block the conversion process.[6] This is one of the biggest reasons why so many people stay stuck in symptoms despite being on thyroid medication. Most of the first-string thyroid medications, such as levothyroxine, replace T4 only. People taking these medications might have enough T4 in their system, but if their body isn't converting it into T3 efficiently, they're not getting the active hormone that fuels cellular function.

The other complicating factor when it comes to conversion is that T4 can *also* be converted into a hormone called reverse T3 (rT3). Reverse T3 works as a buffer to guard against the overproduction of T3 and keeps your T3 levels stable. It also binds to the same cell receptors as T3 does and therefore blocks T3 from working. If reverse T3 climbs too high, it can slow your metabolism and create a host of other problems. Too much reverse T3, which is measured by a blood test, can be triggered by all the same issues that interfere with T3 production in the first place: nutrient deficiencies, elevated cortisol due to stress, poorly regulated blood sugar, bodywide inflammation, and fluctuations in reproductive hormones.[7] Any of these factors can flip the conversion process so that you produce too much reverse T3. In fact, the biggest disruptors of the conversion process are:

- Insulin resistance and elevated blood sugar
- Estrogen dominance (and a lack of progesterone due to perimenopause)
- Low iodine
- Low magnesium

- Low vitamin D
- Chronic stress
- High cortisol
- Genetic variations that impair conversion

We'll dive much deeper into this later in the book because conversion issues and the problem of reverse T3 are two of the most overlooked and misunderstood parts of thyroid health. They are the root cause of why so many people on T4-only medication still feel awful. T3 is like the power switch for your cells, and without it, the lights stay off.

To be and feel truly healthy, your body must be able to convert T4 into T3 efficiently. If this isn't happening and blood testing confirms that you are not converting well or that your reverse T3 level is too high, you will likely need to eliminate T4 and bring in replacement T3 in the form of a prescription pill. When you have enough free T3, your body starts cooperating again.

When Things Go Wrong

As we've seen, thyroid hormones wield tremendous power over almost every aspect of your health. When the thyroid is doing its job—producing the right hormones in the right amounts—and your body is efficiently converting T4 to T3, you live in Optimization Land, where your metabolism, energy, digestion, sleep, and brain all function so beautifully that you never have to think about them. But when your thyroid gets knocked off-kilter—due to hormonal changes, illness, autoimmune issues, or just plain old genetics—it stops your body in its tracks. Hormone production goes wonky, and you end up with one of the following.

Hypothyroidism

Hypothyroidism is a condition in which your thyroid doesn't produce enough thyroid hormone. Production slows down, and everything slows down with it. Energy drops, metabolism drags, and every system that depends on thyroid hormones begins to suffer. You feel drained, heavy, foggy, and flat. Your weight creeps up even though you're doing all the right things. Your digestion slows, your mood dips, and your spark fades. Your hair starts thinning, your skin feels dry, and your mood shifts toward irritability, sadness, or anxiety. Constipation, joint pain, and feeling cold all the time are common. These are the body's ways of waving a white flag, signaling that the command center is losing control.

Fortunately, we have the ability to replace the hormones your thyroid is struggling to make. And when we do it right and truly optimize your treatment, your symptoms disappear.

Hashimoto's Disease (Hashimoto's Thyroiditis)

Hashimoto's disease is the autoimmune form of hypothyroidism. In the big picture, Hashimoto's *is* hypothyroidism, but you can have hypothyroidism without having Hashimoto's. With Hashimoto's, your immune system sends out antibodies that mistake the thyroid gland for the enemy; they think of your thyroid gland as an invader and go to war against it. We don't know why this happens, but it's the same process seen in other autoimmune diseases, such as rheumatoid arthritis, in which the immune system attacks the joints, and celiac disease, in which it targets the villi in your small intestine.

These antibody attacks result in inflammation and gradually reduce the thyroid's ability to produce hormones. If you have an ultrasound, you might see a thyroid that has been beaten up over time. It can look jagged, uneven, or smaller than it should be. In some cases, the gland shrinks so much from this ongoing assault that it barely functions at all.

Hashimoto's is the number one cause of hypothyroidism today, and it is diagnosed by testing for two antibodies, thyroid peroxidase antibody (TPO) and thyroglobulin antibody (TgAb), which show that your thyroid is under attack. Like regular hypothyroidism, it is treatable, and we can replace your missing hormones and get you back to feeling your best. Although it takes time, full remission is possible and your thyroid-attacking antibodies can return to zero.

Thyroiditis

Thyroiditis is simply an inflammation of the thyroid. It can be short term or long term and may resolve on its own, but it's always a sign that something deeper is going on with your body's immune system. Symptoms may include swelling of the thyroid gland and a temporary decrease or increase in levels of thyroid hormone.

Postpartum Thyroiditis

This is the medical term for thyroid dysfunction triggered by pregnancy. The truth is that pregnancy is one of the biggest physical and hormonal stressors a woman's body will ever experience, and it's one of the most common times that thyroid issues appear. Essentially, it's Hashimoto's that was switched on by pregnancy. Puberty, pregnancy, perimenopause, and menopause are the four windows when that autoimmune switch is most likely to flip on. Your doctor will tell you that it will pass and you'll "be fine," but the reality is that this may be an autoimmune condition you need to address.

Hyperthyroidism

This is the other side of the coin, where your thyroid produces *too much* hormone. In this scenario, everything in your body speeds up. Your metabolism burns calories so fast that you lose too much weight at a rapid pace, your heart races, you feel anxious and agitated, you sweat profusely, and you may have muscle tremors or trouble sleeping. Hyperthyroidism is much less common than hypothyroidism, but it is treatable with medication and sometimes surgery, and its symptoms are less easily conflated with other health issues. In this book, I focus on hypothyroidism, the center of the silent epidemic.

• • •

When the thyroid stops leading effectively, the troops lose direction, and every system in your body feels the fallout. Remember, fatigue, stubborn weight, brain fog, hair loss, mood swings, and poor sleep are not random symptoms. They're signals from your command center that it's time to get things back in order.

You Need a Plan, Not Empty Promises

Treating thyroid disfunction in any form is not just about writing a prescription and calling it a day. It's about seeing and evaluating the full picture—TSH, free T4, free T3, reverse T3, the two types of antibodies—and above all, refusing to stop at "normal." It's about understanding that for most people, especially women, "normal" on a lab test means nothing when they still feel like a shell of who they used to be.

Good thyroid care often requires customizing prescriptions for both T4 and T3 and adjusting them regularly. It requires harnessing the often forgotten thyroid hormone T2 to support optimal metabolism and energy. It also requires anti-inflammatory nutrition, hormone balancing, stress support, targeted movement, and nutrient therapy. It's a lifestyle-supported treatment plan, not a one-size-fits-all template.

After completing my functional medicine training, mentoring with the top experts, and earning my doctoral degree, I could have easily jumped onto the wellness bandwagon and sold another trendy "natural thyroid healing" program. I could have built a nutrition plan, listed a few beneficial supplements, and called it a day. But that would have been a lie. I know, both personally and professionally, that healing hypothyroidism and Hashimoto's takes more than just cutting out gluten and meditating; it nearly always requires some form of targeted hormone replacement. You need to partner with prescribing practitioners with excellent training who understand the nuances of this condition. You need a comprehensive strategy, not drugstore supplements. Another elimination diet will not get you feeling like yourself again, and neither will any amount of wishful thinking.

And that's where I come in. I'm here to offer you understanding, direction, strategy—and results.

It all starts with your story, and it's time to get personal. In the next chapter, I'll break down the most common, wacky, and wild symptoms of thyroid dysfunction, how they first appear, and what they tell you about what's really going on beneath the surface.

Chapter 2

Your Body's Loudest Thyroid Distress Signals

Thyroid dysfunction usually starts as a whisper. A little weight gain here, an afternoon energy crash there. Maybe some mild anxiety sneaks in, your hair doesn't feel as thick, your skin starts to feel dry. You brush it off. Must be stress, right?

But then at some point, the whisper gets louder. Suddenly you're twenty or maybe thirty pounds heavier. Your period's a mess. Your sleep is wrecked. Your joints ache. Your focus is gone. You're surviving on caffeine, dragging your body around as though it's made of bricks.

What started as a whisper is now a scream, because you didn't catch the problem early and no one around you knew how to do so. If you're reading this book, you've probably noticed some worrying patterns. Maybe it's the unrelenting fatigue that sleep doesn't fix, the extra weight that seems glued to your body, or the brain fog that turns simple tasks into uphill battles. Or maybe it's the quieter signs, such as mood swings, the kinds of symptoms that get brushed off with "It's your hormones" or "You're just getting older." Does any of this sound familiar?

Thyroid dysfunction can manifest itself in a variety of ways, but the three most common—and often the first—complaints I hear in my practice are weight gain, fatigue, and hair loss. They're the ones that blow up my Just Fix Your Thyroid Facebook group, and they are also the three symptoms that wrecked my life when I was deep in my own battle with thyroid dysfunction. They stole my energy, confidence, and sanity while

I was being dismissed by doctors left and right. I'll cover other symptoms, too, and there are many more—but I'll start here because these are the ones that tend to be loudest and hit women the hardest. Let's explore how and why these symptoms occur and what they can tell us about how your thyroid is performing.

Weight Gain

We're going to be honest here. Weight gain is something that plagues your mind, especially when you're doing everything right and the number on the scale still won't budge. It's one of the most frustrating things a woman can experience: Your weight is going up steadily, and you have absolutely no control over it. You've been trying your best. You've bought ten different diet books, five Instagram-famous weight loss programs, and three "miracle" supplements and even hired a personal trainer.

And still . . . nothing is working.

For women, weight isn't just about health; it's about our confidence, our energy, and our identity. Weight affects how our clothes fit. It predicts whether we want to get dressed to go out with friends. It determines how comfortable we feel getting undressed to be with our partner. It shapes how we show up in the world, and if we even want to show up at all.

And when our bodies start flipping us the bird as the scale goes up again and our favorite jeans don't button anymore, it's all-consuming. From the second we open our eyes in the morning, the thoughts are there:

> *Should I weigh myself today?*
> *No, I don't want to.*
> *I already know the number will be up.*
> *I've been trying so hard.*
> *Why isn't anything effing working?*

This isn't just about vanity, it feels like it's about survival. What you really want is to fit into your clothes again, to feel like yourself again. And if no one else is saying it, I will: It's not your fault. But it *is* your fight.

What Makes Us Fat

Let's start with the truth about fat—and about what gives us a metabolism.

When we hear the word *fat*, most of us think of what we *don't* want on our body. We think about the places it sits and where we see it: on our stomach, on our thighs. And then there is the back fat.

But fat can be both good and bad. Your body needs fat as an energy source. We also need fat to protect our organs, and for warmth. Fat even produces the hormone leptin, which tells our brain that we're full and alerts us to stop eating. Fat itself isn't the enemy—but *excess* fat is.

Excess visceral fat, the kind that wraps around your organs, is dangerous. It's not just about how you look in the mirror, it's about what that fat is doing on the inside. It messes with your liver, clogs your arteries, pumps out cytokines that increase bodywide inflammation, stresses your cardiovascular system, and jacks up your risk of developing diseases such as type 2 diabetes, heart disease, high blood pressure, fatty liver disease, Alzheimer's, and even certain cancers. It slows down your metabolism, throws your hormones out of whack, and creates a perfect storm for chronic illness.[1] While the body positivity movement has been great for helping women reject toxic beauty standards, it is not a pass on ignoring real health concerns.

While the scale gives us a number to obsess over, in reality it's your body fat *percentage*—that is, the ratio of fat in your body compared to muscle, bone, and everything else—that is a much better indicator of your overall health. You can be thin on the outside and if you're out of shape still have a relatively high percentage of body fat. Your fat-to-muscle ratio gives us a picture of how your metabolism is working on a cellular level.

What is metabolism, anyway?

Metabolism is the process by which your body converts molecules derived from food into energy. It is the biological engine behind calorie burning, fat burning, and energy production. When we have a fast, efficient metabolism, our body burns calories around the clock, not only from the food we eat, but from any excess body fat, naturally keeping us slim and energized. But when we have a low, slow metabolism, regardless of how clean we eat, how hard we work out, or how many calories we cut, that sluggish metabolism isn't burning enough fuel. Instead, it stores much of the energy you consume—on your belly, hips, thighs, and anywhere else that loves to hold on to fat.

But here's the truth that most people miss: Your metabolism is controlled by your hormones. It's not a simple "calories in, calories out" equation. Hormones run the whole show. Remember, hormones are your body's chemical messengers, sending signals to your cells to tell them what to do. When it comes to metabolism, they decide whether you burn calories, store them as fat, crash on the couch, or light up with energy.

And when it comes to your weight, the thyroid gland and the hormones it produces, most notably T3, are the master controllers and regulators of your metabolism. If your thyroid is sluggish or underperforming, your metabolism is, too. And that means that calorie burning, fat burning, energy, and weight loss all slow to a crawl, no matter how perfect your eating and exercise plan is.

Let's break down how these beautiful thyroid hormones help keep our metabolism in check.

T3 enters your cells and binds to receptors that stimulate mitochondrial activity, boosting the production of ATP. Remember, mitochondria are the powerhouses of your cells, and ATP is your body's energy currency. The foods you eat are broken down into molecules that are used by mitochondria to create ATP. T3 is like the spark that fires up the mitochondria, and if you don't have enough T3, it's tough to get the fire going. When you have enough T3, your metabolism is constantly humming and your cells are able to burn calories and produce ample ATP all day long. In fact, the presence of T3 helps increase your basal metabolic rate (BMR), which is the number of calories that your body burns in maintaining essential functions, such as breathing and circulation, even when you are at rest.

Although it's often overlooked, T2 also works at the mitochondrial level to ramp up ATP production. Even more impressively, T2 directly promotes the burning of excess fat by converting white adipose tissue—the stubborn fat found on your belly and thighs that serves as storage for excess calories—into brown fat, which is metabolically active and actually burns calories to maintain body temperature and generate heat. T2 appears to increase the number of mitochondria in your white fat cells so that the cells are more like brown fat, a process called "browning."[2] The more brown fat you have, the higher your heat production and the higher your basal metabolic rate. More brown fat activity is also linked to better insulin sensitivity and improved blood sugar regulation[3]—two additional factors in maintaining a healthy weight.

This is why your weight and metabolism are at the mercy of your thyroid, regardless of how often you hit the gym or how few calories you eat. If you're not making enough T3 and T2 or you can't convert T4, your metabolism is turned off, your energy is low, and your ability to burn fat is stalled. To have a metabolism that works well, you need enough T3 and T2 to flip on the switch and fire up the mitochondria in every single cell.

But T3 and T2 aren't the only hormones that have a direct impact on fat burning and metabolism. Insulin, leptin, and testosterone also play crucial roles in healthy weight maintenance across all ages and both sexes. However, their beneficial activity can be short-circuited by poor thyroid performance. If your thyroid levels drop, these hormones will fail you also. Let's take a closer look at the interplay between your thyroid and the other hormones that burn calories and make sure the pounds stay off.

Insulin

Insulin is a hormone produced by your pancreas that is released into your bloodstream every time you eat. Its job is to regulate incoming blood sugar, or blood glucose, by signaling to your cells to take in the glucose to be used as energy. Once your cells have had their fill, any extra glucose is stored elsewhere in the body as fat. When your metabolism is working well, your cells take up and use most of the circulating glucose efficiently, leaving only a modest amount for storage.

Insulin resistance is a condition in which your body's cells become less responsive to insulin. When this happens, it's as though your cells no longer fully hear the messenger, and they stop taking in glucose as effectively as they should. This means that more glucose is left circulating in your bloodstream, which your body then stores as fat. Instead of using what you eat for fuel, your body becomes a hoarder, locking those calories away as it tries to bring your blood sugar levels back to normal. The pancreas then starts overproducing insulin, trying as hard as it can to get your cells to respond. But if your cells are ignoring it, insulin works against you. Essentially it becomes a hormone that promotes fat storage—and that's the last thing you need when you're trying to maintain a healthy weight.

Insulin resistance can have a variety of causes, including poorly regulated blood sugar, a lack of physical activity, excess body fat, genetics, and elevated cortisol levels (more on this below). But it can also be brought on by hypothyroidism. The drop in thyroid hormones leads to an overall slowdown in metabolism that affects your body's ability to use glucose effectively. Too much glucose is left circulating in the bloodstream, which leads to an overproduction of insulin, which in turn leads to your cells' developing insulin insensitivity. Studies show a strong correlation between insulin resistance and hypothyroidism, which together compound your struggle to lose weight. Insulin resistance has also been shown to be linked to other problems, most notably and recently Alzheimer's disease.[4] In fact, Alzheimer's is now being called type 3 diabetes because of how closely it is linked to insulin resistance and poor metabolic health.

Today, most people know that a high-carb, high-sugar diet will spike insulin, or at the very least that a high-carb, high-sugar diet will cause weight gain. But I see many patients in my clinic who are eating ketogenic or are on a strict carnivore diet with low to no carbohydrates and are still gaining weight. Their thyroid signaling is off, so their metabolism is off, and insulin is working against them, regardless of their diets. I tell them: It's not the food, it's your thyroid. The same goes for people who are taking glucagon-like peptide-1 (GLP-1) receptor agonist medications such as Ozempic or Mounjaro but aren't seeing results. GLP-1 medications were designed for type 2 diabetics, and they work by slowing gastric emptying, curbing appetite, and improving insulin sensitivity. But they rely on your metabolism being at least somewhat functional. If your thyroid is underperforming and you are low in T3, your cells are locked in a metabolic stall: no fat burning, no energy production. And even powerful GLP-1s can't override that.

My patient Barbara came to us weighing over 250 pounds. She was a lifelong diabetic, and she was already on a GLP-1 medication prescribed by her endocrinologist, but it wasn't affecting her weight. She had also been diagnosed with a thyroid issue, but it was being treated with T4 medication only. Her blood sugar remained high, and no one could figure out why. But when we finally added T3 and T2 to her treatment plan and got her onto the right thyroid protocol, her metabolism was able to reboot, she reversed her diabetes, and she dropped over one hundred pounds. That's the power of treating the root issue, and in her case, the root was thyroid.

If you believe or know that you are insulin resistant and your thyroid also isn't running at full speed, chances are that your body is in fat-storage mode. The good news is that by fixing your thyroid, we can reverse your insulin resistance and get your metabolism working again. There are also readily available supplements, such as the plant-based chemical compound berberine, that can be helpful in promoting insulin sensitivity and supporting better glucose metabolism (see chapter 9).

Testosterone

After T3, my second-favorite hormone is testosterone, because it's the get-shit-done hormone. It gives us drive, motivation, brainpower, and the ability to build and hold on to muscle. It improves cardiovascular health, balances lipids, stabilizes mood, and revives libido. It also plays a huge role in metabolism.

Despite what most people think, testosterone isn't produced only by men. Believe it or not, it's one of the primary hormones in women, too. Truthfully, testosterone deserves its own book. But for now, here's what you need to know: Testosterone is essential for good metabolic health and hormone balance, especially as we age. It's the third player in the metabolism game, right alongside thyroid hormones and insulin. It improves blood sugar regulation by enhancing insulin sensitivity, boosts the functioning of mitochondria, and helps stimulate the breakdown of stored fat. It's also what determines whether time in the gym translates into actual results, because it directly promotes muscle growth by activating satellite cells in your muscles that repair and grow muscle tissue. It also promotes the protein synthesis necessary to increase muscle mass and strength. On the flip side, it inhibits the effects of catabolic hormones such as cortisol, which can break down muscle tissue.[5] Without testosterone, building and maintaining lean muscle becomes almost impossible, no matter how heavy your weights or how perfect your macros are.

And let's be clear: Muscle isn't just about aesthetics. Muscle is metabolically active tissue. That means that it's a primary driver of your basal metabolic rate, helping you burn fat even at rest. The more muscle you have, the better your metabolism works. Muscle is your organ of longevity. And testosterone is what protects it.

Studies have shown that hypothyroidism also impacts your testosterone level. In women, testosterone is made primarily in the ovaries, which are highly sensitive to any abnormalities in thyroid hormone. Lower thyroid hormone also leads to lower levels of sex hormone–binding globulin (SHBG), a carrier protein made by the liver that binds to testosterone and plays a crucial role in regulating its availability throughout the body. When your thyroid levels tank, all too often your testosterone levels tank, too.

And if your testosterone level is low, you feel it! You get walloped by fatigue, brain fog, weight gain, muscle loss, and low sex drive—all the stuff that so many midlife women complain about. Here's what to watch for.

- You're working out but not seeing results—no muscle growth or body composition changes.
- Your strength is declining or your recovery time is getting longer.
- You feel like a zombie; your energy is tanked, your motivation is gone, and your mood is flat.
- You're gaining fat, especially around the belly, even if your eating habits haven't changed.
- Your libido is MIA, and it's not just a "stress" thing.
- You're constantly tired, even after sleep.
- Your confidence and drive are lower (testosterone is a confidence hormone just as much as a muscle hormone).
- You're dealing with brain fog and have trouble focusing.
- You have dry or thinning skin, brittle nails, and even depressionlike symptoms.

If you're thinking, "That sounds exactly like thyroid symptoms," you're not wrong! Low-testosterone symptoms and hypothyroid symptoms overlap. That's why, in my experience, so many people are misdiagnosed or only half-treated. They take thyroid meds but still feel off because no one has checked their testosterone level. They're still dragging, and they still can't lose weight or build muscle. When it comes to thyroid hormones and testosterone, it's often not a case of either/or; it's both.

Here's another truth: Conventional testing for testosterone is garbage. The "normal" lab ranges are so wide and outdated that they keep both men and women feeling sick and undertreated. To complicate matters further, testosterone is classified as a Schedule III controlled substance, right alongside opioid painkillers. Let that sink in for a second: A natural hormone your body *needs* to function is regulated as though it's dangerous or addictive. And because of its Schedule III status, many doctors are hesitant to prescribe it. Some won't even test for testosterone unless you practically beg. And if you're a woman asking for it? Good luck. You'll likely be dismissed, told that your symptoms are "just aging," and offered an antidepressant instead. You're left without answers and without treatment—all because a hormone that could change your life is locked behind outdated, fear-based regulations.

I firmly believe that testosterone isn't dangerous, it's life giving. I have seen it successfully replace medications such as antidepressants, sleep aids, and even statins. It can save marriages by improving physical and emotional connections on both sides. And it can be the missing piece of the puzzle when it comes to regaining energy and shedding pounds. With my patients, I watch for the interplay between hypothyroidism and testosterone very closely. Sometimes testosterone is what it takes to kick your metabolism back into gear.

Leptin

The next hormone that demands attention when we're talking about stubborn weight and a body that seems to be working against you is leptin. Leptin is your "satiety hormone." It tells your brain, "We're full, we're good," so you don't eat all day long without a pause.

Ironically, leptin is produced by white adipose tissue, or fat cells. But if you think about it, this makes sense: If you have more fat cells, you will release more leptin, which is the body's natural mechanism for slowing caloric intake and moderating weight gain. The release of leptin is triggered by insulin, which, as we've seen, is released by your pancreas in response to high blood glucose after a meal. Leptin's primary receptors are in the brain's hypothalamus, where it helps you decide to stop eating.

Leptin deficiency is rare. Far more common is leptin resistance, which, similar to insulin resistance, occurs when your brain cells stop responding to the hormone's signal. In this case, your brain isn't getting the message that you're full, and you keep eating because your satiety switch is broken. Leptin resistance often shows up alongside insulin resistance and can be a result of hypothyroidism. The elevated levels of TSH associated with an underactive thyroid increase circulating leptin levels,[6] which cause the brain's receptors to become less sensitive to the hormone's effects over time.

If you're dealing with leptin resistance, it's going to show up in some pretty frustrating ways. If you find yourself battling food noise, constant cravings, or the relentless pull toward sugar and carbs, leptin resistance might be at play. These are the red flags.

- You're always hungry even after eating a full meal.
- You constantly crave sugar or carbs, even when you know you "shouldn't."
- You never feel full, no matter how much you eat.
- You gain weight easily, especially around the midsection.
- You feel out of control around food, as though the "off" switch is broken.
- You think about food constantly; i.e., the food noise never shuts up.
- You've hit a weight loss plateau, even though you're doing all the right things.
- You feel sluggish, inflamed, puffy, and as though your body is stuck in fat-storage mode.
- Your energy dips hard, especially in midafternoon, and you're constantly reaching for snacks or caffeine to push through.

Leptin resistance is sneaky because it doesn't just affect your appetite, it also disrupts your brain, metabolism, and ability to feel normal around food. But it's not a lack of discipline. It's a hormone-signaling issue.

A lot of these symptoms look *just like* insulin resistance. And *just like* hypothyroidism. That's because often they're all connected. If your T3 is low, your leptin signaling is disrupted. And if your insulin is chronically high, your leptin is chronically high, which leads to resistance to both. The end result is the same: cravings, fatigue, intractable weight gain, and a less-than-stellar metabolism.

Unlike low testosterone, leptin resistance is not treated with a magic pill. Treatment starts with addressing insulin resistance and correcting T3 level. There aren't any specific supplements for leptin resistance, but compounds such as berberine that can help manage insulin resistance make a difference for many people. From there, treatment focuses on thyroid optimization to make sure you have enough active T3 in your system to regulate everything downstream.

If you are in that frustrated place where nothing works and the scale will not budge, your thyroid may very well be to blame. In my experience, weight gain is the symptom that most people won't tolerate, the red flag that finally pushes them to seek help, even if they've ignored other symptoms for years. It's the cry that breaks through all the other rationalizing, the "I'm just getting older" or "I've been under stress." Too often, that cry is your thyroid asking for help.

But I can promise you this: When you have enough T3 and T2 in your system, you will no longer gain weight even though your diet has not changed. I have been exactly where you are, and I know what it feels like to be free of that cycle. With my thyroid back in balance, my weight is stable and I can enjoy life again. I can have a glass of wine. I can treat myself to that brownie. I can even partake of the occasional sweet potato fries cooked in less-than-ideal oil. And I don't gain weight.

That is the beauty of thyroid optimization. That is what happens when you finally have enough active thyroid hormones doing what they are meant to do.

Fatigue

We all know what being tired feels like. You pull an all-nighter studying for school. Your baby's been crying through the night. You messed up a project at work or you're an athlete who dropped the ball at the ten-yard line, and it's playing on a loop in your head. Such moments interrupt our sleep and lead to fatigue the next day. That kind of tired makes sense.

But low-thyroid fatigue is a whole different animal. It's an exhaustion you can't explain unless you've lived it. It's the kind of fatigue that doesn't go away with a nap or a good night's sleep. The kind that starts to define you and steal your days. And we need to recognize this, because not all fatigue is created equal.

There's a normal kind of tired. You wake up groggy, hit "snooze" a few times, and rely on coffee just to feel human. That kind of fatigue usually points to something being off: Maybe your cortisol is low in the morning, maybe you're not getting deep, restorative sleep, or maybe stress is stealing your energy. We've all been there. It's not ideal, but it's manageable.

Thyroid fatigue isn't just needing a latte to get yourself moving. It is full-body, bone-deep exhaustion. Your muscles feel like concrete. Your brain feels as though it's swimming in molasses. Even your *eyeballs* feel tired. It's the kind of fatigue that makes the simplest tasks feel impossible. No amount of caffeine touches it, and no nap fixes it. And if your thyroid is underperforming, this kind of fatigue becomes your new normal until you finally get the right treatment.

When thyroid fatigue starts creeping in, it also exacerbates other problems. You do what anyone would do to try to fix it: You start eating more often. You grab sugar at midday for a little jolt. You grab a Red Bull here, maybe a 5-Hour Energy drink there. This of course wreaks additional havoc on your metabolism. Just as with weight gain, you start scrolling Instagram, buying energy protocols, trying new supplements, and diving down rabbit holes of "fatigue fixes." You'll try anything. But nothing works.

Thyroid fatigue hits you at the cellular level, destroying your days. It makes simple things such as showering, cooking, or even sending a text feel impossible. Socializing is a mountain you can't climb. By 2:00 p.m., you stare longingly at your couch, hoping you can sneak in a nap. And even if you do, it doesn't help.

The reasons why take us back to science. Thyroid hormones are critical for metabolism, but they're just as critical for overall energy production. Remember, every single cell in your body has a receptor site on it for T3. That means your thyroid isn't just controlling your metabolism, it's also dictating whether your cells are awake and functional. In particular, your mitochondria need T3 to produce ATP, your body's energy currency.

If there's no T3 or not enough of it, your mitochondria can't produce ATP. And if you're not producing ATP, you have no energy. Without T3, your cells are offline. You're not burning fuel and you're running on fumes, and eventually, you run out.

A State of Human Hibernation

There's a fascinating emerging concept in medicine called human dormancy syndrome (HDS), and it's exactly what I've been seeing and describing in the thyroid world for years. Researchers are now recognizing that in some people, the body can enter a state that mimics hibernation. Everything slows down. Metabolism drops. Energy conservation, rather than expenditure, becomes the main priority.

The term *human dormancy syndrome* was coined by Dr. Michael Powell, who described a specific process for diagnosing and treating this state. In his work, which is protected by a US patent,[7] HDS is defined by one key measurement: an elevated ratio of reverse T3 (rT3) to free T3 as compared to that in healthy individuals, combined with clinical signs of slowed metabolism. Those signs include chronic fatigue, fibromyalgia-like muscle pain, obesity or stubborn weight gain, insulin resistance, depression, memory decline, and other dementia-like symptoms. The patent even compares this condition to a hibernation-like state, in which the body reduces energy output to conserve resources, just like animals do in winter.

In other words, HDS is your body flipping the metabolic "off" switch, the result of thyroid disfunction. When your T3 is low or your reverse T3 is elevated and blocking the action of T3, it's as though your body throws a biological circuit breaker. You stop the flow of energy and instead enter survival, or dormancy, mode.

Picture a bear in winter: Its thyroid output slows; its digestion slows; its body temperature drops; physical activity is nonexistent. The bear's body is doing exactly what it's supposed to do to survive long stretches without food or movement. Now translate that to a human who's not producing or converting enough T3. They can't sleep eighteen hours a day in a cave, but their body doesn't care; it's still in shutdown mode. So even though they try to push through the day, they feel like a zombie. They're exhausted, foggy, and stuck.

If someone comes in and tells me they're experiencing deep, unrelenting exhaustion paired with weight gain, brain fog, sluggish metabolism, joint pain, and muscle aches . . . that person is in hibernation mode. That's human dormancy syndrome in real time. It is a metabolic hibernation state, one that won't resolve until their thyroid is optimized and their T3 level is brought back to where it belongs.

Now, not all fatigue means you're hypothyroid. Even in my clinic, we go through a full checklist before arriving at a conclusion. We look at your nutrition, sleep habits, and alcohol intake. We look at your levels of B vitamins, iodine, and vitamin D, all of which are crucial for energy. But when you've been doing this long enough and sat across from thousands of exhausted humans, you learn how to discern someone with a simple nutrient deficiency from someone whose body is in hibernation.

Here's the best part: There's a fix. You have to test and not just guess, but restoring T3 levels, addressing conversion issues, and bringing down reverse T3 will stop the hibernation response. Energy and brain function are usually the first symptoms to improve once thyroid hormone levels are optimized. Your cells wake up. Your mitochondria flip back on. You start making ATP. And that unbearable, bone-deep fatigue starts to lift.

What About Cortisol?

If you're wondering why I've been talking about energy and fatigue and I haven't brought up cortisol, don't worry. You've probably seen cortisol mentioned in every blog post, podcast, and reel about "adrenal fatigue" that tout getting your cortisol just right as the answer to what ails you. Cortisol matters, to be sure, but it has been turned into a scapegoat for every symptom under the sun.

Cortisol does play a critical role when it comes to energy and me-

tabolism, and there *is* a direct link between cortisol and thyroid function. Cortisol is your body's fight-or-flight hormone, produced by the
adrenal glands and released in response to physical and emotional
stressors such as exercise, illness, and fear. Cortisol's job is to prepare
you for battle and survival. It raises your heart rate and blood pressure and increases your blood sugar level so that you have plenty of
glucose available for your cells to use to generate energy. It also has
powerful anti-inflammatory effects that are helpful in case of injury
or illness, and it works with your circadian rhythm to help you wake
up in the morning.

Cortisol is essential, but prolonged high cortisol levels in your body
due to chronic stress can actually create serious problems. Too much
cortisol can fuel bodywide inflammation, which has been linked to autoimmune disorders, heart disease, and cancer.[8] The cortisol gurus online
will also tell you that it can lead to so-called adrenal fatigue, a condition in which your overworked adrenals stop producing enough cortisol,
which causes symptoms such as tiredness and brain fog. In reality, however, these symptoms likely stem from another side effect of too much
cortisol: hypothyroidism.

Cortisol and your thyroid have a bidirectional relationship: A high
cortisol level brought on by chronic stress can disrupt thyroid function
by reducing TSH and hindering the conversion of T4 to T3.[9] Conversely,
your cortisol level can be elevated *due to* low thyroid function stemming
from other causes, which can lead to reduced clearance of cortisol from
your body. Either way, your cortisol level is elevated, which isn't good—
but that doesn't mean that cortisol alone is the root of your fatigue, brain
fog, or extra pounds.

Some adrenal-focused influencers and practitioners push the idea
that if you just "heal your adrenals," your thyroid will follow suit like
magic. They'll tell you to sip on adrenal cocktails, take an adrenal glandular, meditate, do breath work, cut stress, and *boom*, your T3 production will skyrocket and all will be well. I only wish it were that easy.

While the adrenal glands are vitally important, we can't just take a supplement or do an "adrenal reset" and expect our thyroid to magically wake up and start pumping out active T3. That's not how human biology works.

Here's what *is* true: Your adrenals and thyroid talk to each other. They're both part of the endocrine system, yes. But if your T3 is tanked, if your reverse T3 is elevated, if you're on the wrong thyroid meds, undertreated, or not treated at all, no amount of adrenal healing is going to fix it. Those remedies might help *support* your healing process, sure. But they're not the root solution.

You don't fix a broken engine by changing the windshield wipers. And you don't fix hypothyroidism by focusing only on cortisol. Real adrenal burnout isn't just about feeling tired or needing an extra cup of coffee to get through the afternoon. True adrenal collapse usually follows major trauma: divorce, the death of a loved one, job loss, or anything else that bombs your nervous system. I had a patient who lost her child in a drunk driving accident, went through a painful divorce, and got laid off from her job all in the same year. Her adrenal glands weren't just stressed; they were obliterated. Not surprisingly, her thyroid hormones had also tanked. Her system had fully crashed. That's what adrenal burnout looks like.

But most people aren't dealing with full-scale adrenal collapse. What they often have is mild dysregulation: a little too much cortisol in the morning or not enough in the afternoon. What's worse is that many of the symptoms being blamed on the adrenals, such as fatigue, weight gain, brain fog, anxiety, and poor sleep, are coming from an underperforming thyroid.

Cortisol can push up your glucose. It can interfere with T4 to T3 conversion. And it can absolutely make fat loss more difficult. But it's not the first fire we put out. The smartest move is to optimize your thyroid hormones first. That one shift supports your entire endocrine system and hormonal landscape, including your adrenals, so everything else can start to stabilize.

The thyroid needs to be fixed first. Then, and only then, will the other pieces start to fall into place.

Hair Loss

You start noticing hair in the shower drain, and you think, "Hmm, that's new." After you see it for days and weeks, you pick up the clump and count the hairs. It seems like there are more than there should be. So you change your routine a little. You order special shampoos that promise thicker hair. You start washing your hair less frequently. Maybe you try collagen or a hair growth supplement. But nothing works. Weeks pass, and now you avoid washing your hair because it's become a traumatic event. You have five half-used hair growth serums under the sink, every hairbrush in your house looks as though a small gerbil lives in it, and you own a drawer of clip-in extensions you once swore you'd never use, but now you don't leave the house without them.

There was a time when I lived this scenario. I counted the hairs on the shower floor. I'd look down and panic, wondering if I was going to have anything left. The hair I did have wouldn't grow past the tops of my shoulders. It just stalled. It got dry. It broke halfway down the shaft. The texture changed. The shine was gone. I started wearing every kind of extension available: clip-ins, tape-ins, hand tied, keratin bonds, you name it. I've had the cheap ones, and I've had the expensive ones that stay in for two months and cost a fortune.

Hair loss is emotional. It's frustrating. It chips away at your confidence. We all want long, thick, shiny hair like the Pantene Pro-V model in the wind tunnel has, and it's not just a "cosmetic" issue. It's not just about how you look; it's about how you feel about *you*.

I've had patients bring me bags of hair, hoping that if they can show someone how much they're losing, maybe someone will finally take them seriously. And let's be clear: This type of hair loss isn't normal, it's a sign that something in your body is off. And very often, that something is your thyroid.

To be fair, hair loss isn't caused only by thyroid dysfunction. It can be brought on by illness, trauma, or any other type of shock to your system, and many women experience heavy hair loss after pregnancy. But when a notable jump in hair loss comes hand in hand with other classic thyroid symptoms such as weight gain, fatigue, constipation, brain fog, cold hands and feet, and/or low libido and your thyroid labs are anywhere outside of optimal, we can point the finger straight at the thyroid.

In addition to playing a crucial role in metabolism and energy production, your thyroid impacts your hair growth cycle. I say "cycle" because your hair doesn't just grow endlessly. All the hair follicles on your head go through three distinct phases: the *anagen*, or growth, phase; the *catagen*, or transition, phase; and the *telogen*, or resting (and eventual shedding), phase. When you and your hair follicles are healthy, this cycle allows for a naturally regenerative, continuous renewal of hair. The anagen phase is the longest, with follicles remaining active for years. At some point, each follicle detaches from the blood supply, rests for a period, and sheds its old hair. After a few weeks, a new hair begins to grow. If you have a normal, healthy scalp, approximately 85 to 90 percent of your hair follicles are in the active anagen phase, while the remaining 10 to 15 percent are in the resting telogen phase. Believe it or not, most of us shed up to a hundred hairs daily even when our hair is growing just fine.

Your thyroid's role in all this is to help regulate the hair growth cycle by influencing hair follicle development, which in turn affects the length of the growing phase. Thyroid hormone also stimulates the production of hair matrix keratinocytes, the cells that form the hair shaft and structure. If your thyroid is underactive, the normal hair cycle slows to a crawl, and instead of remaining in the anagen phase, your follicles stall out. Your hair becomes thin, brittle, and dry and stops growing past a certain length. And when your follicles do finally reach the telogen phase, they shed fast, and you lose hair every time you shower, brush your hair, or even touch your head.

But the problem goes deeper. If you have Hashimoto's disease, because of its autoimmune aspects, your gut function is likely compromised, too. One of the lesser-known but incredibly common side effects of Hashimoto's is low stomach acid, especially low betaine HCl.[10] This means that you're not breaking down your food properly. You're not extracting amino acids from protein, and you're not absorbing key hair growth nutrients such as zinc, biotin, selenium, and iron. So even if you're eating a perfect diet, your body isn't getting what it needs to build healthy hair. No nutrients to the hair follicles means no growth. Your follicles are starving.

This is why, even after your thyroid hormones are optimized, I often recommend that my patients take a high-quality digestive enzyme with betaine HCl along with enzymes to help them break down protein, carbs, and fats. Because until you fix your digestion, you're not going to fix your nutrient absorption. And until you fix that, your hair won't fully bounce back. But once we calibrate your thyroid hormones and support these downstream processes, your body will remember how to grow hair. These days, my hair is fuller, healthier, and stronger, even if it isn't exactly as it was in my twenties before my hypothyroidism diagnosis. But rest assured: With the right treatment protocol, you *can* stop the shedding and make peace with the mirror again.

The Autoimmune Escalation

If you've been following me on social media for a while or listening to my podcast, you've heard me say this: Autoimmune begets autoimmune. Autoimmune conditions tend to multiply, which means that when we see one autoimmune disorder, we almost always see more.

Since 95 percent of hypothyroidism is caused by Hashimoto's thyroiditis, an autoimmune disease, you're likely already on the autoimmune spectrum. And studies show a statistically significant link between Hashimoto's and alopecia areata,[11] another autoimmune disorder in which your body's immune system mistakenly attacks your hair follicles and destroys them at their root. Alopecia is not your average shedding; whole sections of your scalp stop producing hair entirely, leaving you with patchy bald spots. The follicles are so damaged, they're basically dead.

Once those follicles are gone, it's difficult to bring them back. A topical serum or biotin supplement won't come close; instead, we're talking about going to lengths such as hair transplants, stem cell therapy, platelet-rich plasma (PRP) injections, and other deep-dive treatments. So if you think you may have Hashimoto's, early testing and treatment are essential. We want to catch your thyroid dysfunction before it gets to this point, because the right combination of hormone replacement and nutritional supplementation can stop shedding and save your hair before it's too late.

Other Wacky and Wild Symptoms of Thyroid Dysfunction

In addition to the Big Three—weight gain, fatigue, and hair loss—thyroid dysfunction can spawn other strange effects. These are the lesser-known, often ignored, and most medically gaslit symptoms of hypothyroidism—the ones you might not hear about as being connected to your thyroid, but once someone mentions them, you instantly say, "Yep, that's me."

These symptoms may not be incessantly impacting your self-esteem, like weight gain, or make getting though your workday difficult, like fatigue. They might not be a secret worry that you're reminded of every time you look in the mirror, like hair loss. But they *are* impacting your quality of life in quiet ways. And often, no one, not even your doctor, makes a connection about the cause.

Brain Fog

This is a troubling line I often hear: "I feel like I'm losing my mind." And it's not hyperbole. I've had forty-five-year-old patients share that they are convinced they have early-onset dementia because their mother or grandmother had it, and now they are walking into rooms and forgetting why, searching for words, fumbling in conversations, and losing track of everything from car keys to their kids' schedules.

Maria was one of them. She came in terrified. Her memory was slipping. Her brain felt as though it were stuck in quicksand. She couldn't focus at work or remember simple tasks. She was convinced that

Alzheimer's had begun. But it wasn't Alzheimer's, it was low T3, the active thyroid hormone that, as we've seen, supports memory, focus, concentration, and other brain functions.

Here's an astonishing fact: There are more T3 receptor sites on the brain than anywhere else in the human body. If not enough active thyroid hormone gets to those sites, your neurons will literally not fire or connect to each other properly. You'll be forgetful. Fuzzy. You'll feel as though you're sleepwalking through your life, struggling to grab on to thoughts that refuse to come into focus. It's as though you're looking at the world through a haze.

But here's the good news: When you optimize your thyroid function, the fog lifts. Maria's brain came back online in weeks—not because of a miracle drug but because we gave her body the hormone it had been screaming for.

Temperature Intolerance

Thyroid dysfunction messes with your body's thermostat, but not always in the way you may think. Most people associate low thyroid with feeling cold all the time. And this is common. I've had patients who wear winter coats in July and quietly sneak over to the thermostat at friends' houses and crank it up to 75 degrees because they just cannot get warm.

But here is what most people—and most doctors—get wrong: You can also run hot or be heat intolerant and still be hypothyroid. Most practitioners assume that if you are hot, sweaty, uncomfortable, and peeling off layers in a freezing-cold conference room, you must be hyperthyroid—meaning that your thyroid is overproducing hormones—or simply perimenopausal. But that is often not the case. Low thyroid can also make you heat sensitive, because when your thyroid is underperforming, your body's temperature-regulating system—which includes the hypothalamus as well as your skin, sweat glands, and even muscles and fat, which generate heat through metabolism—is out of sync. The hypothalamus is your body's thermostat, and if it isn't getting the right hormonal signals, your body does not respond to environmental changes the way it should.

I know this firsthand, because I am the one who is always warm. I hate summer. In hotels, I have been known to hijack the thermostat and override the governor so I can drop the room temperature to 65 degrees or lower. That is the only way I can sleep. My friends and family hate coming over to my house because they know they will need a sweatshirt. I always tell them, "You can get warmer by throwing on another layer, but I cannot cool off unless I strip down and stand outside in the snow."

Whether you are shivering in a cardigan when it is 85 degrees or melting while everyone else is comfortable in jackets, the problem can be your thyroid. To be clear, I'm not talking about hot flashes that last a few minutes; I'm talking about constant temperature dysfunction that follows you around all day, every day. With menopause, hot flashes occur because your brain's hypothalamus is thrown off by the decline in estrogen. But similar symptoms can result when your hypothalamus is hit with either too much *or* too little thyroid hormone.

Heat intolerance is one of the most overlooked symptoms of thyroid dysfunction because it does not fit neatly into the typical thyroid narrative. But if you have felt this kind of nonstop internal chaos, you are not imagining it. This is not about mindset or mental toughness; it is about your thyroid's sending faulty signals to every cell that regulates heat and energy. It is your body crying out for help in the only way it knows how.

Again, the good news is that once you start treating the root cause and optimizing your thyroid function, these signals can normalize. Your thermostat can reset, and your body can finally restore the temperature balance it has been missing.

Depression and Anxiety

Hypothyroidism has a huge impact on mood. If I had a dollar for every patient who was handed an antidepressant instead of a proper thyroid panel . . .

Here is how it usually goes: You tell your doctor that you feel tired and foggy or that you are anxious and not sleeping well, and they suggest an antidepressant from the selective serotonin reuptake inhibitor (SSRI) family such as Prozac, Lexapro, or Zoloft. Or if you say that you've lost your get-up-and-go, that you feel disconnected from everything, and that your motivation is low, they call it depression and send you out the door with another pill, telling you to check back in six months.

What is missing? A requisition for free T3 and reverse T3 testing. No one stops to question whether your brain chemistry feels off because your thyroid is off.

Persistent feelings of anxiety, lethargy, apathy, or moodiness, although they can mimic depression, are not always due to a serotonin deficiency; they might be due to a T3 deficiency. Thyroid hormone plays a surprisingly large role in brain chemistry, helping regulate neurotransmitters related to mood and motivation such as serotonin, dopamine, and gamma-aminobutyric acid (GABA).[12] If your thyroid is underperforming, your brain does not have what it needs to regulate your mood properly. Antidepressants don't help because the root cause goes untreated.

My patient Sarah came to me after being on antidepressants for over ten years. She told me, "I never really felt depressed, I just felt like I wasn't myself anymore." Her doctors kept adjusting her dose, switching her medications, and telling her to be patient. Not once did anyone run a full thyroid panel. When we finally tested her free T3 and reverse T3, the problem was obvious: Her T4 was not converting properly. Once we optimized her thyroid hormones, her mood lifted, her energy returned, and for the first time in over a decade she was able to come off the antidepressant medication.

The T3–Mental Health Connection

Most people, including plenty of doctors, never think to connect your thyroid and your mind. Yet researchers have known for decades that thyroid function and mental health are deeply intertwined. If you have thyroid dysfunction, your chance of developing a mood disorder climbs quickly. Depression, anxiety, and irritability are not minor side effects; for many people, they are the main event, consuming their world and often misdiagnosed or dismissed.

Here's what we know: People with hypothyroidism have a much higher risk of developing a major depressive disorder.[13] This is not limited to those with advanced or long-standing thyroid disease, in which hormone levels are far outside the normal range and symptoms are extreme. Even mild thyroid dysfunction, what's called subclinical hypothyroidism, when your TSH is slightly elevated but your free T4 and free T3 are still in a "normal" range, can trigger persistent low mood, brain fog, and apathy.

Studies show that thyroid hormones, especially T3, have a direct impact on the parts of your brain that regulate emotion and stress resilience, such as your hippocampus and amygdala.[14] When your T3 is too low, those areas of your brain can't function properly. Your nervous system gets stuck in a sluggish, depleted state that no amount of talk therapy or positive thinking can override.

This is why assessing thyroid function is so important for anyone grappling with depression. Research has found that correcting thyroid dysfunction can lift mood symptoms that nothing else has touched.[15] In some cases, adding T3 to an antidepressant regimen has been the turning point after years of feeling stuck. T3 is not a stimulant. It does not artificially rev you up. It simply gives your brain the hormone it has been starving for.

I see it in my practice every week. Patients come to me with a diagnosis of depression or anxiety and a long list of medications they have tried. They have been told that they are "treatment resistant" or that something is permanently wrong with them. Meanwhile, they're cold all the time, dragging themselves through the day, battling crushing fatigue, and wondering why they cannot think clearly or feel like themselves.

But once we start treating their thyroid, especially by restoring T3, they feel something shift. They don't wake up the next morning singing show tunes and skipping down the street, but they start having glimpses of themselves again. Their energy begins to return, the mental fog starts to lift, and the constant heaviness in their mood eases. They realize that the problem was never just "in their head"; their thyroid was at the center of it all. This is not rare, it is just rarely recognized.

Frozen Shoulder and Other Musculoskeletal Problems

I bet you never thought that joint-related issues could be directly connected to your thyroid, but your frozen shoulder may not be a result of that extra round of burpees or your CrossFit workouts. Frozen shoulder is when your shoulder joint suddenly stops moving the way it used to. Maybe it hurts when you reach behind your back to unhook your bra, or you can't lift your arm more than 90 degrees without wincing. Most people chalk it up to age, injury, or their long-standing love of side sleeping. But in fact, the cause could be your thyroid.

Frozen shoulder, also called adhesive capsulitis, presents as pain, stiffness, and a shoulder joint that feels stuck. Your shoulder joint capsule, the connective tissue sac that surrounds the joint where your shoulder blade and upper arm bone meet, becomes inflamed, thickens, and tightens, leading to restricted motion until it is almost locked in place. On the surface, this looks like an orthopedic issue. But in reality, it could be tied to your endocrine system.

Believe it or not, endocrine disorders, especially thyroid disease, are strongly linked to frozen shoulder. If you have hypothyroidism or Hashimoto's, your risk of developing this frustrating condition is nearly three times higher.[16] Many people spend months in physical therapy, doing endless stretches and exercises for their shoulders, but nothing improves because the real issue is not being addressed.

Thyroid hormone plays a major role in regulating how your body builds and breaks down connective tissue. When your thyroid levels drop, your system can't maintain healthy turnover of collagen and elastin, the primary proteins that form the structure of all connective tissue. Instead, your tissues start to accumulate excess proteins, which leads to swelling. Over time, this thickens the shoulder joint capsule, creating an environment that behaves more like scar tissue than like healthy tissue. Your shoulder joint is literally being suffocated on a cellular level.

But this isn't just about the tissue itself, it's also about inflammation. If you have Hashimoto's thyroiditis, your immune system lives in a state of chronic low-grade inflammation. The inflammatory signals don't just stay in your thyroid; they circulate throughout your entire body, landing in joints and soft tissues where they don't belong. Even a minor strain or repetitive motion can set off an exaggerated response. Your immune system overreacts, ramps up the inflammation, and refuses to switch off. This is why frozen shoulder often shows up without any obvious injury.

Uncontrolled or undertreated hypothyroidism makes the situation worse. One frozen shoulder can easily turn into two. Your range of motion can shrink more and more over time, and the longer you stay in a low-thyroid state, the harder it is to regain full function without major intervention.

I've had patients walk into my office convinced that they had a sports injury or repetitive strain issue, only to discover that their thyroid was the real culprit. Their reverse T3 test results come back sky-high, their free T3 is scraping the bottom, and no one has ever connected the dots. Their shoulder pain turns out to be one more clue that their thyroid has been neglected for years.

Frozen shoulder is only part of the picture. Low thyroid function can slow down nerve conduction, dull your reflexes, and stiffen your muscles.[17] You might feel tingling in your hands and feet, burning pain, numbness, or heaviness or even have balance problems that you can't explain. When your nerves start to misfire, your muscles stop working the way they should. And when that happens, your joints and the rest of your musculoskeletal structure pay the price.

If your shoulder suddenly locks up and there is no explanation, do not just blame your workouts or your pillow. Take a closer look at your thyroid labs. Your shoulder might be telling the story your doctor has been missing.

Constipation

The smooth muscles of your intestines have receptors for T3, which means that thyroid function and gut function are interconnected. In particular, thyroid hormone plays a role in gastrointestinal motility, the rate at which food moves through your intestines. A lack of T3 will slow down peristalsis, the coordinated contractions that move the food along, which can lead to—no surprise—constipation. If you're suddenly blocked up even though constipation has never been an issue before, your thyroid could be to blame. Conversely, a too-high T3 level can accelerate motility, leading to poor nutrient absorption and diarrhea.

But the links between gut health and thyroid health don't stop there. A healthy gut microbiome produces enzymes that facilitate the conversion of T4 to T3, and a poor gut microbiome—one with fewer beneficial bacteria and an overgrowth of harmful ones—creates an inflammatory environment that can reduce the production of these enzymes.[18] Poor gut health also reduces the absorption of key nutrients such as selenium, zinc, and iodine that are essential for thyroid hormone production—one more reason why eating clean and taking supplements and probiotics to support your gut is a worthy investment in your long-term health.

Luckily, constipation is one of the easiest symptoms to resolve with proper dosing of T3. With your thyroid optimized, you'll be regular again before you know it.

Allergies

Thyroid disorders often come with a heightened histamine response or an increased risk of seasonal allergies to things such as pollen and grass, as well as new food allergies or food sensitivities. This is especially common with Hashimoto's. Your immune system is already on overdrive, confused and swinging a sword at everything it sees, so it makes sense that pollen, perfume, or even your cat can suddenly set off a reaction that has never happened before.

There appears to be a particularly strong correlation between allergic rhinitis (including hay fever) and Hashimoto's.[19] When I first met my client Erin, she wasn't just sneezing in the spring, she was sneezing at everything—dust, mold, her parents' dog—all year round and living on Claritin and Benadryl just to function. Once we optimized her thyroid, her immune system calmed down, the constant inflammation eased, and her sinuses opened up. She still takes a Claritin now and then when the pollen count spikes, but she no longer reacts to every little trigger in her environment. It's not that her allergies disappeared; it's that her thyroid optimization helped regulate her immune response so her body could handle the world around her again.

If you suddenly find that you are experiencing allergies that you never had before, along with other suspicious symptoms, your thyroid, not the grass and flowers in your front yard, just might be the culprit.

Migraines

Many people think that migraines are just "in their head," both literally and figuratively. Maybe it's stress, maybe it's your hormones, maybe it's just your genetics, right? Well, yes. And also no.

Migraines can absolutely be tied to sex hormone imbalances, especially low estrogen or progesterone. And they can be triggered by certain foods, light, sleep deprivation, or sensory overload. But if you have hypothyroidism or Hashimoto's and you're also getting migraines, your thyroid might be at the root of it all.

A study recently reported in *Frontiers in Neurology* found that individuals with hypothyroidism are more likely to experience migraines than those with normal thyroid function.[20] The researchers concluded that thyroid dysfunction may play a role in both the development and the persistence of migraine attacks. This connection also shows that thyroid hormones don't just support and enable brain function, they also influence how the nervous system processes pain and inflammation. When your thyroid is out of balance, those pain pathways can become overactive, making migraines more frequent, intense, and difficult to treat with standard approaches.

Why? Because your thyroid hormones regulate vascular tone—the state of contraction or relaxation of your blood vessels—and nervous system stability.[21] If your thyroid is sluggish, your blood vessels can overreact, triggering the cascade of inflammation and constriction that ends with you curled up in a dark room with a cold washcloth over your face.

Another study found that Hashimoto's thyroiditis is surprisingly common in people with migraines.[22] In this analysis of nearly a thousand migraine patients, over 11 percent were also diagnosed with Hashimoto's. This points to a strong autoimmune link, not just a hormonal one. It suggests that the same immune dysfunction that attacks the thyroid can also drive inflammation in the nervous system, setting the stage for migraines that become harder to control over time.

When thyroid function is optimized, a lot of people who have suffered from migraines see them disappear. I have seen patients go from living on daily migraine meds such as Imitrex to never thinking about migraines again. Weekends are given back. Life is given back. And no, it was not because they started meditating or switched to gluten-free crackers. It was because we got their thyroid working properly again.

Dry Skin

Patients come to me with dry skin that no lotion can soothe. Thyroid hormones regulate skin cell turnover and the moisture production of your skin's eccrine glands, and if your levels are low, your skin cells shed more slowly, and you are left with dry, itchy, flaky skin no matter how much you moisturize. You can slather on all the Aquaphor you want, but unless you treat the underling hormone imbalance, you won't regain the smooth, soft skin we all want.

Thinning Eyebrows

Many women with thyroid dysfunction experience thinning or loss of the outer third of their eyebrows. It's straight out of the thyroid dysfunction playbook, yet it still flies under the radar in most conventional medical offices. Eyebrow loss usually accompanies hair loss, and it is caused by the same autoimmune response that attacks the hair follicles on the scalp. Fortunately, as with other hair, your eyebrows will come back most of the time once your thyroid hormone levels are optimized.

. . .

In addition to the symptoms listed here, it's possible that you have noticed other strange, small changes in your body that aren't on any checklist. Could they be due to low thyroid? Yes, it's possible. In my experience, when thyroid imbalances are treated properly, a lot of people see weird, seemingly unrelated symptoms disappear.

So I'll leave you with this: What you feel is real. Trust yourself and what you know about your body. You don't have to have every textbook thyroid symptom to know that something is off. Your job is to notice, track, and speak up when your body is waving a red flag. Above all, you do not have to settle for being told that it's just stress, it's just hormones, or that it's all in your head. It isn't. It's real. Optimize your thyroid, and you might just be shocked at what else falls into place.

Chapter 3

How Did I Get Here? Understanding Triggers and Risk Factors

O ne of the most common questions I get is "What's the root cause of my thyroid problem?" My answer usually surprises people. In many cases, the thyroid itself is actually the root cause of everything else going wrong. When your thyroid is not working, every other system that depends on it starts to break down.

Take the brain, for example. As I said, there are more T3 receptor sites in the brain than anywhere else in the body. If your thyroid is low, you might feel anxious or depressed, not because you are lacking Prozac or Wellbutrin but because you are lacking thyroid hormone. The real root cause of your mood disorder could be your thyroid. The same is true of your metabolism. If you have gained weight and can't seem to lose it, even with clean eating and consistent workouts, low thyroid function is a likely culprit.

But if we really want to dig deeper into what caused your thyroid to malfunction in the first place, we need to unpack that step by step.

Science has shown that about 95 percent of all hypothyroidism is autoimmune related, usually in the form of Hashimoto's thyroiditis. And when it comes to understanding autoimmune conditions, I always like to reference the work of Dr. Alessio Fasano, a professor at Harvard Medical School and the author of seminal books on celiac disease and gluten intolerance. He describes autoimmune disorders as being like a three-legged stool[1] (I love this analogy because it breaks down auto-

immune diseases into something you can clearly visualize and understand), as follows.

Leg One: Genetic Predisposition

The first component of any autoimmune disorder is genetics. I always
ask my patients, "Did your mom, grandma, aunt, or sister ever have a
thyroid problem?" Nine times out of ten, they'll say, "Oh, yes, my mom
and grandma were both on Synthroid."

When I ask, "Did they have Hashimoto's?" the answer is usually
"No, they were never told that." But then they'll mention something
like rheumatoid arthritis, which is another autoimmune disease. Here
is what I can tell you: The odds of both your mom and grandma having
primary hypothyroidism—that is, hypothyroidism *not* linked to any
type of autoimmune activity or disorder—is extremely low. Primary
hypothyroidism is relatively rare and usually caused by things such as
chemotherapy, radiation, certain medications such as beta-blockers,
severe nutrient deficiencies, or direct trauma to the thyroid gland.
Hashimoto's, on the other hand, has a strong genetic component, just
like other autoimmune diseases. It can run rampant in families, especially in women, since we are more susceptible to autoimmune conditions in general. In most cases, it is far more likely that someone in
the patient's family tree had undiagnosed Hashimoto's and passed that
genetic tendency down the family line to where it is now showing up in
the patient's own labs.

Leg Two: Leaky Gut

The next leg of the autoimmune stool is leaky gut. This one is spoken about
less but is just as important. Leaky gut syndrome is a condition in which
the lining of the small intestine becomes more permeable, allowing larger
molecules and bacteria to pass into the bloodstream. Your gut lining is
meant to be a tight barrier. But over time, thanks to the poor quality of
the soil in which our food is grown, processed foods, and the chemicals,
pesticides, and toxins in your makeup, hair products, body lotions, and

even on your furniture and carpets, your gut lining takes a hit. When it breaks down, tiny, toxic bacterial components called lipopolysaccharides (found in the outer membrane of gram-negative bacteria) slip through and enter the bloodstream, triggering immune responses.[2]

Almost all of us are walking around with some degree of leaky gut. It's simply a result of the world we live in. But for people predisposed to autoimmune disorders, in which the body's immune system goes into overdrive and attacks itself, having a leaky gut is like opening the floodgates. Your body is forced to contend with additional toxins and in doing so lays the groundwork for a scenario in which your immune system spirals out of control.

Leg Three: A Trigger or Stressor

The third leg of the stool is the trigger, an illness or event that flips the autoimmune switch to the "on" position. It could be something completely natural, such as pregnancy, during which your hormones fluctuate wildly. Or it could be perimenopause or menopause, which causes another hormonal roller coaster. It could also be something environmental, such as living in a moldy home or having your mercury fillings improperly removed and replaced. Emotional trauma can be a trigger too: caregiving, divorce, the death of a loved one, or a job loss. Sometimes it's a viral or bacterial reactivation such as Epstein-Barr virus or Lyme disease. Sometimes it's a mystery. But once that switch is flipped, it doesn't turn off on its own. The immune system goes into overdrive and turns on the body itself—and often, for reasons we don't fully understand, on your thyroid.

Realistically, even when we do figure out what the trigger was, there's usually no way to undo it. We can't un-have a baby. We can't stop perimenopause from happening. We can't stop your body from aging. We can't go back in time and remove the trauma or prevent the virus from entering your system.

What we can do is offer your immune system support, lower your inflammation, and optimize your thyroid function to stop symptoms from taking over your life. Because once the switch is flipped, it's not about reversing the trigger, it's about treating the thyroid dysfunction left behind.

The Most Common Environmental Triggers

I know you love going down the "root cause" rabbit hole, so let's go one step farther, shall we? The reality is that many aspects of modern life just aren't good for our bodies or our thyroids. But too few medical practitioners are connecting the dots between thyroid damage and lifestyle factors such as environmental toxins and even some standard medical treatments. Some of these factors are more avoidable than others, but if we don't educate ourselves and start paying attention to what we're putting into and on our bodies, we might as well just accept a lifetime of being fat, foggy, and fatigued. These triggers are real. They might not be obvious, and they're rarely talked about in mainstream medicine, but they matter. And many are avoidable if you know what to look for.

If you have thyroid problems in your family history or even if you have already received a hypothyroidism diagnosis, there are steps you should consider taking to minimize any ongoing environmental stress on your thyroid. Here are some of the most consequential thyroid disrupters that you will want to be aware of.

Environmental Toxins

I've already mentioned environmental factors, such as pollution, mold, and everyday chemicals, as triggers for flipping on the Hashimoto's switch or contributing to leaky gut. But what about the direct impact of environmental pollution on the thyroid itself? Environmental toxins are some of the most significant drivers of thyroid dysfunction, and not enough people in the medical space are talking about it.

When my husband and I moved to Iowa about three years ago, I immediately started noticing the planes. They flew overhead almost daily, spraying pesticides and herbicides over the cornfields just over a mile from our home. I could see them out my window, looping and swooping, leaving long white chemical trails behind. It wasn't just one field or one season a year; it was constant. Those chemical sprays were being dumped into the air around us.

One of those sprays was glyphosate, a herbicide widely used all over the world on nonorganic grains and produce. Glyphosate disrupts your endocrine system, wrecks your gut microbiome, contributes to leaky gut, and binds to essential minerals such as iodine and selenium, both critical for healthy thyroid function.[3] Some studies even suggest that it can directly block the enzymes needed for thyroid hormone production.[4]

Here's what I do know: You don't have to live next to a farm to be exposed. Even though the planes were over a mile away, the residue, drift, and legacy of those chemicals still reach all of us. They settle into the air we breathe, the soil beneath our feet, the water we drink, and even the food we think is safe. Organic or not, nothing is completely untouched. This stuff infiltrates everything. It gets into our lungs, bloodstream, and cells. And we're all exposed to it every day, at one level or another.

And it's not just glyphosate. We're hit with a chemical cocktail daily. There are bisphenol A (BPA) in plastics, phthalates in cosmetics, flame retardants in furniture, perchlorate in drinking water, and heavy metals such as mercury and cadmium in the soil. These toxins disrupt hormone production, block thyroid receptors, and can even trigger autoimmune conditions such as Hashimoto's. Let's take a look at some of the worst offenders and how they can derail your thyroid health.

The Toxic Three

Halogens are a group of elements defined by their particular molecular structure. Iodine is a halogen, and I touched on its critical role in thyroid function and overall health in chapter 1. We absorb iodine all the time through dietary sources such as fish and dairy products, and it can even be taken as a supplement to assist in treating thyroid disorders. But the other three halogens that we are exposed to regularly—fluorine, chlorine, and bromine—are highly toxic. Fluorine is a gas at room temperature, so we encounter it mostly in its halide form: fluoride. Because of their similar chemical structures, all these nasty little disruptors compete directly with iodine in your body and can wreak havoc on your thyroid function.

As we saw in chapter 1, iodine is an integral component of thyroid hormone, and your thyroid gland needs iodine to be able to synthesize T1, T2, T3, and T4. But if any of the other three halogens are present in your body in high enough concentrations, they can displace iodine and prevent it from being absorbed by your thyroid and used for hormone synthesis. Instead, your thyroid mistakenly absorbs the toxins. And if you're flat-out deficient in iodine, guess what wins every time? These three toxic halogens get in, take up shop, and start wrecking your body, leading to everything from hypothyroidism to broader hormonal disruption to cancer.

Fluorine/Fluoride

Still brushing your teeth with fluoride toothpaste? Then stop. Just stop. It's 2026. We're done pretending that fluoride is helping us. You've probably already had a lifetime's worth from those fluoride treatments at the dentist's office. While small amounts may help prevent cavities, the reality is that fluoride is toxic to the body, especially the thyroid.[5]

In 1945, our government decided to put fluoride into the public water supply as a way to strengthen kids' teeth and prevent decay. For decades, however, it has been ignoring data showing that fluoride exposure is linked to reduced IQ, especially in boys.[6] More than a lack of fluoride, it's the daily onslaught of "Frankenfoods" that are high in sugar and bathed in colored dyes that are ruining our teeth. We can do a lot to prevent cavities just by eliminating the garbage in our diet.

If you have a family history of thyroid disease or are currently undergoing treatment for hypothyroidism, I believe that you would do well to avoid fluoride. It is a known thyroid disruptor.[7] Yet most of us are still putting it into our mouths, just inches away from our thyroid gland. Every. Single. Day.

Chlorine

It's in our tap water. It's in our bathwater. It's in swimming pools. It's what we've used for decades to kill bacteria in water systems. But when we drink chlorinated tap water, shower in it, swim in it, or use unfiltered water for cooking, we absorb it.

Chlorine is found in 98 percent of public water systems in the United States, and it's not just a disinfectant, it's a toxin. Like all other halogens, it competes directly with iodine in your body and can therefore disrupt and impact your thyroid function. It also disrupts your gut health, leading to—you guessed it—leaky gut.[8] So every time you drink tap water at a restaurant, get ice from the fridge, or take a long, hot shower without a proper filtration system, you're exposing your thyroid to potential damage.

Were you a swimmer in high school? Did you, like me, grow up spending a lot of time in the pool? Did you live at your local rec center every summer? If so, you've already been exposed to more chlorine than you realize.

I have functional medicine colleagues who swear by using iodine supplements to protect their kids before they head to a chlorinated public pool. They make sure their children have iodine in their systems ahead of time so their thyroids are already "occupied," which helps block the toxic chlorine and prevent it from entering the vulnerable gland. If you're battling thyroid issues, that's a smart move.

Bromine/Bromide

Bromine is another toxic halogen used in industrial production, and it's everywhere. It's in your clothes, carpets, rugs, car interior, and countless plastics, including the packaging of just about every processed food on the market. It is widely used as a flame retardant in textiles, and certain dyes contain bromine to increase their stability and persistence. Like chlorine, it can be used as a disinfectant for hot tubs and spas. Its halide form, bromide, was widely used in dry cleaning and even in medicine as an anticonvulsant until concerns about its toxicity led to its replacement by safer, more environmentally friendly options. Even so, bromine is still out there, even if most of us have never heard of it. And the more exposure you have to it, the larger the hit your thyroid takes.

Avoiding Environmental Toxins: The 80/20 Rule

When it comes to protecting and supporting your thyroid, I recommend the 80/20 rule and live by it myself. Essentially, the 80/20 rule says: There will always be 20 percent of toxic exposures that you can't control. And that's okay. Maybe that 20 percent comes from where you work. Or that shampoo you really love. Or the city you live in. That's life.

On the other hand, you *can* control what goes into and is put on your body about 80 percent of the time. You're going to need to change some things if your health matters to you. I'm not about to tell you to toss all your body wash, shampoo, and makeup, because no one wants to do that. That's not living, and I wouldn't want to do that, either.

Let's say you're on a road trip. You're stuck at a gas station in the middle of nowhere, and your only water option is bottled water in plastic. You know that the water has been chlorinated and "purified" with other chemicals, and you know that bottle is likely made with bromine and other toxins. Guess what? You drink the water in the plastic bottle or you dehydrate. You're not going to die from one bottle. Give yourself grace.

The same goes for food. Unless you want to grow all your own food in your backyard and never set foot in a restaurant again, there will always be things in your diet that you can't 100 percent control. And that's okay.

My goal is to help you feel better while recognizing that you're a human being doing your best to survive and support your body and thyroid in the chemical shitstorm that is modern life. So do your best to follow the 80/20 rule. Control what you can. Let the rest go. You don't need to obsess over every toxin in your bathroom cabinet or find a hairdresser who uses all-natural hair dye that turns your hair pumpkin orange. And if your perfect MAC concealer happens to have a few questionable ingredients, wear it anyway and rock it.

I'm not always going to tell you what you *want* to hear, but I'll be darn sure to tell you what you *need* to hear. And sometimes what you need is the relief of knowing you don't have to be perfect. Even small adjustments help.

Toxic Medications

I want to talk about another major player in the thyroid disruptor game: medications. Before you protest, let me explain. Yes, medications are designed to help us, and the vast majority of them *do* help. Many of them are medically necessary. They can save and prolong our lives well beyond what our ancestors enjoyed just a few generations ago. So this is not about jettisoning medications that you need to keep you living a healthy, high-quality life (and I would absolutely put thyroid medications into that category). But if we're talking about triggers, certain medications can have a negative impact on your thyroid. It's important to be aware of these potential side effects so that you can make informed decisions given your own health history and be attuned to any thyroid changes that may result.

Here are some common medications that can cause problems.

Birth Control

Whether it's "the pill" or a hormonal intrauterine device (IUD), a birth control method that introduces synthetic hormones into your body can play a role in thyroid dysfunction. Ninety-five percent of women have used birth control at some point in their lives, and a 2021 study found that women who had taken the pill for more than ten years were nearly four times as likely to develop hypothyroidism.[9] The science isn't settled, but what we do know about how birth control works and how it changes your total hormonal landscape suggests that caution and vigilance are needed when it comes to protecting your thyroid.

What effect does birth control have on your hormones? Honestly, it's not good. Birth control pills shut down your body's natural hormone production. By giving you synthetic estrogen and progestin, they override the signaling of the hypothalamic-pituitary-ovarian axis. That means your brain stops releasing the signals that would normally tell your ovaries to make real estrogen and progesterone. Ovulation never happens, and your natural hormone rhythms flatline.

When you take the pill, you are essentially hitting the "mute" button on the entire communication loop between your brain and your ovaries. Normally, your hypothalamus nudges your pituitary, and your pituitary sends out follicle-stimulating hormone (FSH) and luteinizing hormone (LH), which tell your ovaries to grow a follicle and prepare for ovulation. The accompanying rise and fall of estrogen and progesterone each month is what creates your energy, mood stability, sleep patterns, and even your sense of well-being.

But once you're on hormonal birth control, that rhythm ceases. Your own estrogen and progesterone levels barely move. Your FSH and LH stay chronically low. And over time, this can lower your level of anti-Müllerian hormone (AMH), which is a marker of ovarian reserve. It doesn't mean that you can't ever get pregnant, but it does show that your ovaries aren't being stimulated the way they should be.

Then there's SHBG. Birth control pills increase your level of sex hormone–binding globulin (SHBG).[10] I always describe SHBG as a very sticky train. Hormones jump onto it and hitch a ride. Free testosterone jumps on. Estradiol can also jump on. Even some thyroid hormone can bind to it. And once those hormones are stuck to the SHBG train, they're not free anymore. They're still riding around your body, but they can't get off at the stop where they're actually needed.

So when your SHBG level goes up from the pill, you're left with little to no free testosterone to work with. And that's when women start saying they just don't feel like themselves. They feel flat, disconnected, as though the spark they used to have has quietly disappeared. They can't put their finger on it, but they know that something feels off. And for many women, that "off" feeling starts with the pill binding up their hormones.

But that's only the beginning. Synthetic estrogens also stimulate the liver to produce more thyroid-binding globulin (TBG),[11] which works the same way as the SHBG train. TBG is the train that delivers thyroid hormone to every cell in your body. You need some thyroid hormone on that train for transport, but you also need enough that can jump off when it reaches the destination.

When TBG increases, more of your circulating T4 and T3 get stuck on the train. They are bound up and inactive. They're circulating in your body, but they can't hop off at the designated stop to do their job. So you can have plenty of thyroid hormone in your blood, yet almost none available for use.

High levels of estrogen and synthetic progestins also change the liver enzymes that convert T4 to active T3.[12] They can also increase inflammation, which slows conversion even more. And when conversion slows, it doesn't matter if your labs look "normal." What matters is how much free T3 your cells can actually access.

This is why some women can be on the pill and feel cold, exhausted, irritable, and foggy, and be bloated, constipated, and constantly gaining weight, even when the numbers on paper say they're fine. They're living in a functional hypothyroid state created by synthetic hormones binding up everything they need to function. The pill changes the hormonal landscape in a way that standard lab tests simply don't catch.

Now, let me pause here and say something important. I understand why women go on the pill. I did it, too. For so many women, it's peace of mind around preventing an unwanted pregnancy. And regardless of your religious beliefs or personal views about birth control, it's available to us, and it's a woman's individual choice whether to take it.

I certainly didn't want to get pregnant when I was growing up. I was in high school, focused on my life and my future, then enjoying my college years. I wasn't ready to have a child in my twenties or even my thirties. So yes, birth control absolutely came in handy for me. I wouldn't go back and change that choice, because it protected me and allowed me to live life on my own terms.

I'm not here to judge anyone for choosing hormonal birth control, because I chose it, too. I'm here to make sure you know what it does to your thyroid and your hormones. You deserve the full picture so you can make the most informed decision for your thyroid and your health.

Just please don't take it to avoid having a monthly bleed. Please! I see this often with women in their forties who want to skip the inconvenience of a period. But that monthly bleed tells you that your cycle is functioning. Shutting it off can feel convenient, but it silences a vital feedback mechanism. It keeps you from knowing what is really going on inside your body. It can mask symptoms that would otherwise point you toward a thyroid issue, an estrogen imbalance, or perimenopause.

The bottom line is this: Hormonal birth control isn't harmless. It affects your brain, your ovaries, your metabolism, and your thyroid. You have every right to choose it. You also have every right to understand how it may impact your health so you can make empowered decisions about it at every stage of your life.

Beta-Blockers

Beta-blockers, also called beta-adrenergic blocking agents, are commonly prescribed for high blood pressure (hypertension), heart palpitations (arrhythmia), and sometimes to reduce the heart's workload after a heart attack. They include atenolol (Tenormin), carvedilol (Coreg), metoprolol (Lopressor and Toprol XL), and propranolol (Inderal, Innopran, and Hemangeol).

Some beta-blockers, particularly nonselective ones such as propranolol, can interfere with thyroid function by inhibiting the activity of the enzyme type 1 deiodinase (D1), which converts T4 into T3.[13] Even if your thyroid was working normally before you started taking a beta-blocker, your cells can end up starved for T3. This leaves you with all the familiar symptoms of hypothyroidism, such as fatigue, brain fog, weight gain, depression, cold hands and feet, and low motivation. In fact, beta-blockers are so effective at blocking the production of T3 that they are sometimes used to help manage the symptoms of *hyper*thyroidism, in which the thyroid gland is overactive.

Unfortunately, thyroid dysfunction resulting from the use of beta-blockers often goes undetected because, as we've seen, most conventional providers rely on testing for TSH, and sometimes T4, without testing for free T3 or reverse T3. If your TSH falls within the "normal" range, they may assume that your thyroid is fine, without realizing that your medication is interfering with the activation of your thyroid hormone.

If you are taking a beta-blocker and noticing symptoms that could be thyroid related, it is worth asking your doctor about alternative medications or requesting a complete thyroid panel to determine if the drug is part of the problem.

Chemotherapy and Radiation

Chemotherapy and radiation are lifesaving cancer treatments, but they also come with a cost. Anyone who has undergone these treatments knows that they are major physiological stressors, and often your thyroid takes a hit. Radiation can directly damage the thyroid gland,[14] leading to inflammation, reduced function, or even full-blown hypothyroidism down the line. Chemotherapy floods the body with toxic agents that can interfere with hormone production, either by damaging the thyroid itself or by triggering an autoimmune response that leads to Hashimoto's thyroiditis.

Those of us who have had cancer are not always told to monitor our thyroid afterward, but we should. And we should be reminding our primary care providers that we want it done as part of our follow-up care. Chemotherapy and radiation might be necessary treatments, but recovery is necessary, too, and that includes protecting and supporting your thyroid every step of the way. This means having regular thyroid labs, watching for symptoms of low thyroid function, and giving your body the nutrients and rest it needs to restore a healthy hormone balance. Your thyroid may have taken a hit during treatment, but with the right monitoring and support, you can give it the best chance to recover.

Puberty, Pregnancy, Perimenopause, and Menopause: The Hormonal Roller Coaster

In my practice, major hormonal shifts are the most common triggers of thyroid problems in women. Puberty, pregnancy, perimenopause, and menopause can all flip the switch, and for many of us, that's when everything starts to unravel.

Let's start with puberty. I can't tell you how many women have told me, "Looking back, I think that's when it all started." A young girl suddenly gains weight out of nowhere, even though nothing in her diet has changed. She's tired all the time, she's moody, her periods are a mess, and everyone chalks it up to "just being a teenager." The surge of estrogen during puberty can unmask an underlying thyroid issue that's been quietly brewing.

After we make it through the hormonal changes of adolescence, the next big hormonal shift for many women is pregnancy. While pregnancy is certainly a natural state, it's also a massive stressor on the body. Your hormones surge, your immune system self-suppresses, and your metabolism kicks into high gear to support your growing baby. For some women, their body never recovers. I hear it all the time: "After my first child, my body went to Hell in a handbasket." They never lost the baby weight, their hair started falling out, their energy tanked, and postpartum depression sometimes made an entrance. All of it gets brushed off as "new-mom life," but what's really happening to many of these women is that their thyroid was pushed to the breaking point. Postpartum thyroiditis and Hashimoto's are incredibly common and almost always missed in the shuffle of pediatric checkups and sleepless nights.

Perimenopause and menopause are another story—and one we'll dive into more deeply in the thyropause chapter. But I'll tell you this: These are the years in which symptoms of all kinds slam women the hardest. Progesterone drops first, estrogen swings wildly, and by the time menopause hits, both hormones are on the floor. In many women, that roller coaster leaves the thyroid gasping for air, but they are told that it's just "aging." No, it's your thyroid waving the white flag.

The bottom line is this: Major hormonal transitions aren't small blips on the radar. They're earthquakes, and they are a part of being female. If your symptoms began or got worse during or after one of these life phases, it's not in your head. These are some of the most common triggers I see, and the sooner we connect the dots, the sooner you can stop blaming yourself and start getting answers.

Thyroidectomy or Radioactive Iodine Treatment

If you have been diagnosed with thyroid cancer, surgery may be required to remove the cancerous portion of the thyroid gland, and sometimes the entire gland must be removed to eliminate all traces of the cancer. Surgery may also be warranted if you have a large goiter or thyroid nodule that is impairing your thyroid function or visibly protruding from your neck. These surgeries can be lifesaving, but often no one talks about the bigger picture: what happens afterward. Because we're not just talking about removing your appendix or some other random piece of tissue—we're talking about your thyroid, the gland that helps run your entire body. If you take it out, you'd better have a plan for keeping your body balanced afterward, and all too often people don't.

Radioactive iodine (RAI) is used to treat thyroid cancer by way of a pill. Your thyroid loves iodine; it soaks it up like a sponge. When you take the radioactive form, the gland grabs onto it, and it destroys the cells from the inside out. But there's a catch: RAI doesn't just go after the cancer cells. It doesn't leave the "good" tissue alone; it wipes out everything, and that's the point. RAI treatment is often chosen because in theory it's easier on you than surgery—no incision, no scar, no anesthesia. But often the result is the same as with surgery: Your thyroid is so damaged that it might as well be gone. And does the radiation stay confined to just the thyroid, or is it released into your body? The honest answer is: We don't know.

Here's what all too many doctors get wrong after thyroid surgery or treatment with RAI: Most of them will prescribe you just T4. That's it. Just T4. No T3, even though your entire thyroid has been wiped out.

And in my opinion, that is negligence. Because your thyroid doesn't just produce T4 and T3, it's also one of the sites outside the liver and the gut where T4 to T3 conversion happens. If you give a patient only T4, it's like crossing your fingers and wishing on a rainbow that somehow the patient's body, without a thyroid gland, is going to be able to convert enough synthetic T4 into enough active T3 to fuel every single cell in her body.

This is why so many of the women I see experience persistent or even *worse* symptoms of hypothyroidism after surgery or treatment with RAI. The surgery, which was designed to fix one problem, actually triggers another. My firm belief is that every person walking around who has had a full or partial thyroidectomy or RAI treatment should be on some form of T3. Period. End of story. Even more than that may be required, such as T2 or nutritional supplements, to get you optimized. Having surgery or RAI treatment doesn't necessarily mean that your thyroid problems are over and done; sometimes it is just the first step in an ongoing journey back to thyroid health.

You don't go through major surgery or the radioactive destruction of your thyroid just to feel worse. You can thrive after these treatments, but you have to fight for it. In parts II and III of this book, I'll show you how.

Thyropause or Menopause—or Both? The Overlap That Leaves Women Gaslit and Unheard

---

As you cross into your forties, the lines between symptoms of thyroid dysfunction and perimenopause or menopause begin to blur. Overlapping symptoms may arrive at the same time, and to make diagnosis even more challenging, they look and feel the same to you. If you're a woman dealing with both thyropause and menopause, low thyroid and declining sex hormones, it's a double whammy. A hormonal landslide.

The first thing my patient Christina said to me when we sat down at her first appointment was "Dr. Amie, I'm fat, and I'm hot all the time." I chuckled a little inside, because I'd been in her shoes. The weight gain and heat intolerance were all too familiar. You can't get cool when this kind of heat takes over. You're burning up while people around you are comfortable. For me, it was thyroid related. But now that I'm in my fifties, like so many other women, I'm feeling it from the menopause side, too. Heat intolerance suddenly becomes full-blown hot flashes and night sweats.

Christina was forty-nine years old and a successful, respected nurse practitioner. But energywise, she was barely making it through the day. It had started about a year before, and she told me that no matter how much or how well she slept at night, her energy was flagging. On top of the fatigue, she was seeing expansion around her midsection—something she assumed was a result of falling estrogen. "My body has just shifted," she said. "My clothes got tighter. My skin looks ten years older. Sex with my husband? No, thank you . . . my libido is kaput. I don't even feel like myself. And worst of all," she went on, "I used to love my work. But now I don't have the mental clarity or the motivation to dive into patient care. If I can't figure out what's going on with me, how can I help anyone else?"

We followed the same process we use with every patient in my clinic. First, I listened—really listened. I gave Christina the time and space to voice her concerns, ask questions, and express her fears without being rushed or dismissed. Then I reassured her that the symptoms she was experiencing weren't random. Many of them were connected, and we were going to get to the root of them. So we tested. Because in my clinic, we don't guess, we test. Every time.

Her labs told the full story: Both menopause and thyropause were wreaking havoc. Her reproductive hormones—estradiol, progesterone, and testosterone—were nearly nonexistent. Her follicle-stimulating hormone (FSH) and luteinizing hormone (LH) levels were elevated. She hadn't had a period in ten months, and while the textbook definition of menopause is twelve consecutive months without a menstrual cycle, I don't believe in waiting for a calendar to confirm what the body is already screaming.

To top it all off, her fluctuating hormones had triggered Hashimoto's thyroiditis. Her labs revealed high levels of thyroid peroxidase antibody (TPO) and thyroglobulin antibody (TgAb), which confirmed that her immune system had begun attacking her thyroid. Antibodies are like the soldiers of the immune system, and in Christina's case, they had launched a full-on assault. Her immune system thought it was protecting her, but in reality it was destroying the gland she needed to function, which only made her menopausal symptoms worse.

This is the definition of what I call thyropause: the moment in your forties or fifties when your thyroid gland short-circuits and seemingly implodes due to your fluctuating hormones. Your reproductive hormones and thyroid hormones spiral downward at the same time, creating an avalanche of debilitating symptoms that leaves you feeling wrecked and desperate for answers. Unfortunately, perimenopause and menopause are all too often the catchall excuse for women's health troubles. And because the symptoms of menopause and thyroid dysfunction are extremely similar, the thyroid piece gets overlooked and dismissed all the time.

Menopause on its own is no joke, and I firmly believe that hormone replacement therapy should begin the moment a woman hits perimenopause and continue seamlessly through menopause and beyond. However, in many cases, this needs to be done while *also* treating thyropause. Until you address both, you won't stand a chance of regaining your former energy and vitality and feeling like yourself again.

Thyropause: The Missing Piece of the Puzzle

It's a beautiful thing to see the spotlight finally shining on menopause. Everywhere you turn, there seems to be another book or another expert interview, podcast, or news article dedicated to the topic. That's progress! Women deserve honest conversations about what happens as their bodies age and real solutions for how to manage and replace their declining hormones during menopause with hormone replacement therapy.

But for all the noise and new information, I believe that an essential component is missing from the conversation. Almost every single one of these discussions leaves out the thyroid, and I don't think it's possible to talk about menopause without addressing the thyroid's role. The reverse is true as well—you can't talk about thyroid function without talking about menopause. They are intertwined in a way that most clinical experts have not yet recognized. The question I hear all the time is: Which came first, thyropause or menopause? And the answer is . . . it's complicated.

Your thyroid and your ovaries are in conversation throughout your life. In fact, they have a reciprocal relationship. Your ovaries have receptors for T3, and thyroid hormone is essential for proper ovarian function, influencing everything from your menstrual cycle to your fertility. Low thyroid hormone or hypothyroidism can stop ovulation, lead to irregular periods, and increase your risk of miscarriage during pregnancy. It can fast-track menopause and lead to early ovarian failure. On the flip side, estrogen and progesterone, which are produced by the ovaries, can affect the availability of T3. Estrogen also stimulates the production of thyroid-binding globulin (TBG), the carrier protein that binds to thyroid hormones in your bloodstream and makes them unavailable for use. If your estrogen level is too high relative to your progesterone level—a scenario known as estrogen dominance that is common in perimenopause—you can end up with too much TBG and low levels of free T3.[1] Ovarian cysts are also closely associated with thyroid nodules and hypothyroidism. That's a lot of overlap!

Furthermore, evidence from clinical studies increasingly shows that *any* problems with the hormonal chain of command between the brain and your ovaries—the hypothalamus-pituitary-ovarian (HPO) axis—can spill over and impact the hypothalamic-pituitary-thyroid (HPT) axis, and vice versa.[2] These two lines of communication in your endocrine system are so easily influenced by each other that it's hard to disentangle them—which makes the "Which came first?" question even harder to answer.

Sometimes it's perimenopause that pulls the trigger. In your forties, your progesterone drops first, then your testosterone, then your estrogen. The drop is stressful. Both testosterone and estrogen have anti-inflammatory properties, so when you lose them, you get a rise in bodywide inflammation. And stress and inflammation, as we know, are a recipe for autoimmune reactions. Hashimoto's that was hiding in the background or in your genes suddenly flares up.

Other times, the thyroid has been dragging along quietly for years. Hashimoto's can sit dormant, almost silent, until falling reproductive hormones push it over the edge. It is possible to power through low-grade thyroid dysfunction, but if you ignore it long enough, your whole system tips. Your sex hormones crash earlier than they should, then the thyroid breaks down completely, and the symptoms of full-on menopause hit hard and fast.

Either way, once things start to unravel, it doesn't matter where it began—thyroid or ovaries, Hashimoto's or hormones. When one falls, the rest follow. And you have to treat them all.

Restoring Hormonal Harmony

When it comes to thyropause and menopause, I don't believe that we can look at one hormone or set of hormones in isolation. We cannot achieve correct diagnoses or optimal patient treatment outcomes without an approach that considers everything.

You can't treat sex hormones without treating the thyroid. Period. They go hand in hand. If the thyroid isn't optimized, your body won't be able to properly use any hormones you give it through hormone replacement therapy. We shouldn't be adding estrogen and progesterone to systems that are ill-equipped to metabolize or respond to these hormones and then wondering why women still feel like garbage.

What blows my mind is how many so-called functional or integrative doctors are still getting this wrong. And don't get me started on the pop-up hormone clinics with cheap monthly memberships that lure people in with low prices and false promises. Behind the scenes they're plugging everyone into the same protocol: same hormones, same doses. There's no real testing and certainly no attention paid to the thyroid.

At my clinic, we customize every protocol, dose, and step based on recent tests and data, not only on assumptions or symptoms, and you should demand the same from your practitioner. We never hand over a prescription for estrogen or progesterone cream and send someone out the door without fully understanding what's happening inside their body. In addition to thyroid function and hormone levels, we look at adrenal health, blood sugar regulation, gut function, inflammation markers, and nutrient status—because no hormone is an island, and healing requires a multipronged approach.

Let's break down the hormones involved in menopause to understand just how they overlap with thyropause—and why tackling your symptoms requires a strategy that takes *all* your hormones into account. It's going to get a bit science based here, so bear with me. It's important that you understand how your body works.

FSH and LH

Follicle-stimulating hormone (FSH) and luteinizing hormone (LH) are the brain's direct line of communication to the ovaries. Produced by the pituitary gland, they regulate the menstrual cycle, stimulate ovulation, and direct the production of estrogen and progesterone.

Here's how the feedback system of the hypothalamic-pituitary-ovarian (HPO) axis is supposed to work: At the start of the menstrual cycle, the hypothalamus releases gonadotropin-releasing hormone (GnRH), which tells the pituitary gland to release FSH. FSH stimulates the growth of ovarian follicles, which contain eggs and produce estrogen as they grow. As estrogen levels rise, they stimulate the release of LH, which triggers ovulation. After ovulation, the follicle transforms into a corpus luteum, which continues to produce estrogen and progesterone. The rising levels of estrogen and progesterone provide feedback to the hypothalamus and pituitary gland to stop the cycle until the next one begins.

In a woman with healthy hormone function, FSH and LH rise and fall with the menstrual cycle, directing the production of the reproductive hormones that keep us feeling young and vital. Estrogen rises, progesterone follows, and everything flows the way it should. But when estrogen and progesterone begin to naturally decline during perimenopause, the early signals from the pituitary get louder. FSH and LH levels climb, as if the brain is shouting, "Come on, ovaries, do your job!" The problem is that the ovaries are retiring. They have clocked out, and no amount of yelling by the pituitary is going to bring them back to their full function.

This disconnect—the brain's increasing the volume of its signaling—is what tells us that the perimenopausal shift has started. High FSH and LH levels aren't a problem in and of themselves, just a red flag that reproductive hormone production is slowing down, your body's hormonal landscape is changing, and that bodywide inflammation is on the rise. And when this happens, the thyroid feels it, too.

FSH and LH levels can also be directly affected by the thyroid. Hypothyroidism can induce hypogonadotropic hypogonadism, a condition in which the pituitary gland does not produce enough LH or FSH, which consequently prevents ovulation. This is why we often see menstrual irregularities in younger women with hypothyroidism. Fortunately, when we correct their thyroid hormone levels, their levels of FSH and LH return to normal.

Progesterone

When I met Julie, she was forty-one and exhausted, irritable, and ten pounds heavier than she wanted to be despite clean eating and regular workouts. Her ob-gyn had told her that it was "just perimenopause" and prescribed hormonal birth control. Her primary care doctor ran basic thyroid labs, declared her "normal," too, and wrote a prescription for an antidepressant. But when we dug deeper at our clinic, we found that Julie's progesterone was almost nonexistent and her thyroid conversion was sluggish. She wasn't just in perimenopause, and she didn't just have a thyroid problem. She was in thyropause, too, dealing with that sneaky overlap in which both systems are wobbling at the same time. Once we supported her progesterone and optimized her thyroid, her sleep came back, her mood leveled out, and the weight started to come off.

Progesterone is the hormone that helps you feel calm and steady. It's the one that supports deep, restful sleep, balances your mood, improves insulin sensitivity, and even acts as a natural diuretic, so it prevents bloating and water retention. It also supports your thyroid function by counterbalancing your estrogen and keeping your TBG in check so that you can maintain ample circulating levels of free T3.

Progesterone is the first hormone to taper off in perimenopause, and when it falls, everything shifts. Suddenly you're holding on to water like a camel. Your sleep gets choppy. Your patience is thin. Your emotions run wild. You find yourself snapping more easily, feeling irritable and overwhelmed. It is common for my female patients to say, "Everyone keeps asking me why I'm being such a bitch." And usually they admit, "I don't even know why I'm acting like this." That's low progesterone talking.

This natural decline in progesterone has a direct impact on your thyroid in several ways. First, progesterone plays a role in regulating the immune system and inflammation, and when it drops, inflammation rises. Inflammation, as we've seen, is one of the main triggers of Hashimoto's thyroiditis. A low progesterone level also impairs your ability to convert T4 into T3, so even if your thyroid labs come back "normal," you can still feel miserable. If you already have borderline thyroid function, losing progesterone is like losing the last safety net holding things together.

In truth, progesterone problems can be present in women in their twenties and thirties, long before menopause is even on their radar. Low progesterone during these years shows up as a host of symptoms that you probably chalk up to "feeling hormonal." Heavy periods, painful cramps, anxiety, insomnia, bloating, breast tenderness, and difficulty getting pregnant can all be signs of low progesterone. And as I talked about in chapter 3, taking hormonal birth control suppresses your own natural progesterone production. Sometimes when women go off the pill, their progesterone never rebounds.

By the time a woman enters menopause, her progesterone is virtually nonexistent if she is not replacing it through bioidentical hormone replacement therapy. No progesterone means more inflammation, more sleep disruption, more anxiety, and even more sluggish thyroid function. It becomes a perfect storm: Your thyroid slows down further, your metabolism tanks, diet-resistant weight comes on, and fatigue is your new normal.

Fortunately, replacing progesterone with HRT is a good, relatively simple first step to normalizing thyroid function. Taking progesterone not only reduces the symptoms of menopause, it also reestablishes the hormonal baseline needed to support the T4 to T3 conversion that your body needs to thrive.

Testosterone

At age forty-five, my patient Sarah told me she felt like her edge had disappeared. On the outside, she was keeping up appearances, still working long hours and being successful at her demanding job. But she admitted that on the inside, she was pushing herself through every day and described it as "running on fumes." Her workouts weren't doing what they used to. She was softer and weaker, and no matter how hard she trained, her body didn't respond. Her libido was gone, leaving her feeling disconnected and frustrated in her marriage. When we ran her labs, the reason was obvious: Her testosterone was on the floor, and her thyroid was dragging. In her case, low testosterone wasn't just draining her confidence and energy, it was adding fuel to her hypothyroidism.

As I said in chapter 2, testosterone is my second-favorite hormone to talk about because it really is the "get shit done" hormone. It drives your motivation, sharpens your focus, builds your confidence, fuels your libido, and gives you the strength to build and hold on to lean muscle. Most women don't realize that testosterone is actually our most abundant hormone—even more than estrogen. When it drops, your spark goes with it. Suddenly the energy you used to count on is gone. You're tired and unmotivated, and your body feels softer, squishier, and less well defined. The mental edge you once had slips away, and getting through the day feels like dragging a boulder behind you.

But testosterone does more than help us build muscle or increase our sex drive. Like progesterone, it helps regulate our immune system and tamp down inflammation. When your testosterone level falls, it doesn't just change your mood or your body composition; it can also flip the switch on autoimmunity. That's one reason Hashimoto's shows up so much more in women than in men. Men's naturally higher testosterone level gives their immune system an extra layer of protection that women lose as their testosterone declines.

Testosterone can decline at any age, but it naturally starts to fall after the age of forty in both sexes. Studies show that in women, testosterone can decline by roughly 50 percent between the ages of twenty and forty-five.[3] That's a major shift in your hormonal picture, one that has direct implications for your thyroid. Beyond the increased vulnerability to autoimmune disorders, the drop in testosterone adversely impacts your insulin sensitivity and metabolic health.[4] Because it is harder to build and maintain muscle, your basal metabolic rate slows and your body fat percentage increases. And as we've seen, poor insulin sensitivity and a rise in body fat put direct stress on the thyroid.

The connection between testosterone and your thyroid goes both ways, which means that thyroid dysfunction can tank your testosterone. Low thyroid hormone levels throw off the hypothalamus, which regulates the production of many other hormones, including testosterone. Low thyroid hormones also lead to an increase in sex hormone–binding globulin (SHBG), the protein that binds to reproductive hormones including testosterone and transports it throughout the body. If you have too much SHBG, there is less unbound, free testosterone available for your cells. You can see how this turns into a vicious cycle: Low thyroid function lowers testosterone, low testosterone increases inflammation, and inflammation further damages the thyroid.

The good news is that testosterone therapy isn't just for men. Women benefit just as much when it's prescribed correctly. Bringing testosterone back into range restores energy, strength, focus, and sex drive. Even more, it helps the thyroid by lowering inflammation and quieting autoimmune activity. Sometimes, the testosterone level improves on its own when thyroid function is optimized. But if you need to take proactive steps, they're well worth it. When you replace declining testosterone, you protect your thyroid, brain, muscles, metabolism, immune system, sex life, and overall vitality.

Estrogen (Estradiol)

Before I dive in to talk about this familiar hormone, let's clear something up. When I say "estrogen," I'm not talking about a single hormone. You actually have three different estrogens in your body: estradiol, estrone, and estriol.

Estradiol is the star of the show, the primary female sex hormone produced by your ovaries. It is present in your body in high levels during your reproductive years, with peak concentrations occurring during ovulation. It plays a crucial role in puberty, pregnancy, and your menstrual cycle, and it keeps your mood steady, your brain sharp, your metabolism humming, and your bones, skin, and heart healthy.

Estrone is produced by adipose (fat) tissue, and it is more of a backup supply. It can be converted into estradiol by enzymes, and its level increases after menopause to support cardiovascular function, cognitive function, and bone health as the ovaries produce less estradiol on their own. Estrone is a "growth" estrogen, and honestly, we don't want too much of it because it can overstimulate tissues and increase cancer risk. The third estrogen, estriol, is the weakest of the three and shows up in large amounts only during pregnancy.

When I talk about bioidentical hormone replacement during perimenopause and menopause, I'm talking about replacing estradiol—the queen. Here's why it matters for your thyroid: Estradiol and the thyroid talk to each other. Estradiol helps your cells respond to thyroid hormone, so if estradiol is low, thyroid symptoms often flare even if the thyroid itself hasn't changed. Flip it around, and if thyroid hormones are low, estradiol metabolism slows down. Either way, you get an imbalance. But the biggest problems occur when estradiol *rises* relative to its companion hormone progesterone—a scenario that occurs in perimenopause called estrogen dominance.

During perimenopause, estradiol doesn't ease its way down like a dimmer switch; it's a roller coaster. One day it spikes, the next day it crashes. But progesterone slips away quietly and continually in the background. In a normal menstrual cycle, progesterone and estrogen move together. Estrogen rises and progesterone comes in to steady it, and this rhythm keeps your mood, metabolism, fertility, and everything else working together in perfect harmony. But when progesterone declines during perimenopause, estrogen takes over. And that's how we end up with estrogen dominance—not because there's too much estrogen per se but because there's too little progesterone to balance it. That's when the mood swings, bloating, anxiety, crying spells, and brain fog hit. "Dominant" doesn't necessarily mean sky-high; sometimes the estrogen levels aren't even that high at all. It's just that the ratio is off. And when the estrogen-to-progesterone ratio is off, you feel it.

Estrogen dominance invariably hits the thyroid hard. Not because it shuts the thyroid down directly, but because it changes how thyroid hormones are carried, used, and perceived in the body. High estrogen levels increase the amount of thyroxine-binding globulin (TBG) produced by your liver.[5] As TBG rises, more circulating T4 and T3 become bound and inactive. Total thyroid hormones may look normal or even high, while free T3 and free T4 remain low, or low to normal. This disconnect is one of the biggest reasons why women are told their labs look fine, while in reality they feel anything but.

Estrogen dominance shows up often with oral contraceptives, improperly dosed hormone therapy, and estrogen replacement used without considering the thyroid. In women who are already hypothyroid, a rise in estrogen often creates a higher demand for thyroid hormone, meaning their existing dose is no longer enough. Add in estrogen's effects on immune signaling and thyroid tissue stimulation,[6] and you begin to see why thyroid disorders are more common in women, and why treating hormones in silos never works. When estrogen dominates, the thyroid pays the price, even if on paper it looks like it is doing its job.

Once menopause begins, estrogen dominance is no longer a problem because your estradiol level drops off a cliff. That's when you get the hot flashes, night sweats, vaginal dryness, joint pain, stubborn belly fat, broken sleep, and sharp decline in focus and motivation. You feel as though you're aging at warp speed because in many ways you are. And without estradiol to help your cells respond to thyroid hormone, the thyroid falters, too.

Megan was forty-eight when she came to me. She was married with two kids, and she had a career she had once loved. But she'd been struggling for years. In her early forties, symptoms had started with bloating, anxiety, and mood swings. Her doctor had told her they were "just stress." But they weren't stress; they were estrogen dominance showing up. Her progesterone had fallen, her estradiol was all over the place, and no one had bothered to explain it to her.

By the time she arrived at my practice, she had crashed. Labs showed that her estradiol was almost gone, her progesterone was gone, and her thyroid was crawling. She didn't just feel off, she felt broken. Her brain fog was so thick that she couldn't remember why she'd walked into a room. She cried constantly. She couldn't sleep. Her libido vanished. She snapped at her kids, avoided her husband, and canceled plans with friends. She even googled "mental institution near me" because she thought she was losing her mind.

She told me, "I don't feel like myself anymore. It's like I'm watching someone else live my life. I want to either run away or disappear. I don't care which."

I explained to her that this wasn't "just" anxiety or depression. This was thyropause, and she was in a full-on chemical collapse. Her body had stopped making the hormones that had protected her mood, her brain, her confidence, her sense of self. When your thyroid and your hormones crash together, life unravels. You feel like a stranger to yourself. And the scariest part is how fast it goes from being "a little off" to being "completely unrecognizable."

But here's what I told her: This isn't permanent.

We rebuilt Megan's health from the ground up. We restored her hormones, both estrogen and progesterone. We optimized her thyroid. We gave her body the support it had been missing. And slowly, she came back. Her sleep returned, her clarity came back, the weight started coming off, the tears slowed. She didn't just feel better—she felt like herself again.

Estradiol isn't optional. It's essential. And when it disappears, everything feels harder. Add thyroid dysfunction, and that's when it all collides into thyropause. The symptoms overlap, they fuel one another, and they leave women feeling like strangers in their own skin. It feels as though your body betrayed you overnight, but in fact it wasn't overnight; it was years of imbalance, ignored or tolerated until everything fell apart.

This is why we treat your thyroid and your reproductive hormones together—because when we do, everything changes. Thyroid function is inextricably linked to estrogen, progesterone, and testosterone, and you can't truly optimize one without optimizing all the others.

The Beauty of Bioidentical Hormone Replacement

We are extremely fortunate to live in an age in which science has given women a way to recalibrate their hormones as they get older. Hormone replacement therapy (HRT) has been a watershed treatment in women's health and changed the lives of women everywhere. Depending on your age, you may be years away from needing HRT, or you may need it now. But hear me when I say this: Even if you think your thyroid is the only problem, there may be ways that selective, precisely calibrated HRT for sex hormones can help.

Here's what I want you to know: Bioidentical hormone replacement isn't just about feeling a little better or smoothing out a few symptoms. It is vital for life. These hormones have far-ranging effects and benefits that ripple throughout your entire body. Sure, there are the aesthetic perks we all love, including better skin, stronger hair, a faster metabolism, and an easier time maintaining muscle. These are the things you see and feel almost immediately.

But the benefits run much deeper. Bioidentical hormones also protect your bones, your brain, your breasts, and your heart. They lower inflammation. They improve insulin sensitivity. They help regulate your immune system and keep you resilient as you age. When people say that hormone replacement is optional or just a vanity fix, they are missing the point entirely. Hormones are foundational to good health.

And when you pair bioidentical hormone replacement with thyroid optimization, that is when you see real transformation. This combination is what moves people out of survival mode and back into living fully. It is what brings back energy, vitality, and the sense that you are in your own body again.

That's the true fix, the Thyroid Fix. In part II, I'll show you how to advocate for proper care and achieve its transformational benefits for yourself.

The Fix: Your Plan to Finally Feel Like You Again

Chapter 5

What the Numbers *Really* Mean: Decoding Lab Results

I know that by now you've taken in a lot of information. I hope you've seen your own story reflected in the patient examples I've shared. Now it's time to start looking more closely at *your* story, at the distinct thyroid picture created by your own symptoms, experiences, and lab results.

If you've already had testing and blood work done, this chapter will arm you with the information necessary to understand the results—what they tell you and what might be left unsaid. It's important to know what each marker in your blood work means so that you can connect it to the symptoms you have. If you are at the beginning of your thyroid journey, this chapter explains the labs that can be ordered by your provider and discusses what they do (and often don't) reveal. I want you to know exactly what blood tests to request and why. When you are familiar with these tests, you will be in the best position to advocate for the kind of lab work that can lead to customized—*not* cookie-cutter—treatment and care.

If you're still in the mindset that every word that someone in a white coat says to you is gospel, you might not think it's possible to read or understand your own labs. Maybe you've been told that it's too complicated, or you assume that you wouldn't understand them anyway. But if you keep thinking that you can't interpret your own numbers, you'll stay dependent on someone else to tell you what they mean, even when those interpretations keep you sick.

I developed the material in this chapter to teach you how to decode your own labs. In my public thyroid Facebook group, I see people posting their lab results daily, desperate for someone to tell them what is really going on. They aren't looking for shortcuts; they want the truth. They want clarity. And like you, they want to feel better.

Trust me when I say that it's entirely possible for you to learn to read your own labs. And when you do, you will gain more than just information; you will gain power. You will find your voice. And you'll have the ability to stand up for yourself and ask for the treatment you know you need. You won't have to accept "Everything looks fine" as an answer when you know damn well that nothing feels fine. Because we don't just want to be average. We want to feel f*#$ing amazing!

"Normal" Is a Setting on the Dryer

Before we go any further, I want to talk about the word *normal*. In the medical world, there is an abbreviation used to describe your lab results in relation to a standard lab value range: WNL. Translation: within normal limits.

At first glance, that seems like good news, right? You hear "within normal limits," and you breathe a sigh of relief. You may even feel a flicker of hope. "Whew, okay, good, at least nothing is wrong," you say to yourself. But before you go patting yourself on the back for fitting into the bell curve, let's talk facts.

"Normal" is a setting on the dryer. It should never be used to describe your health. Because as I've said, you don't want "normal," you want *optimal*.

Normal means average. It means you're being compared to the general population, which is not necessarily a pool of vibrant, energetic, thriving people. It's a mix of the tired, the inflamed, the overweight, the medicated, and the chronically ill. That's not the bar we should be using to gauge your health.

Even worse, back in the day, "normal" ranges weren't created by studying healthy humans.[1] They were pulled from blood samples taken from people in hospitals: people who were already sick, people dealing with diabetes, heart disease, depression, autoimmune conditions, cancer—you name it. When your doctor says, "Everything looks normal," what they're actually saying is "You're in the same range as this group of unwell people we used to define normal." Knowing this, "normal" may not be something to celebrate.

Here's an example. In the United States, labs such as Quest Diagnostics and Labcorp set the "normal" range for thyroid-stimulating hormone (TSH) anywhere from about 0.4 to 4.5 mIU/L, or even up to 5.0 mIU/L. That number is deemed to be universal, regardless of whether you're a twenty-five-year-old woman, a fifty-five-year-old man, or an eighty-year-old nursing home patient. It's the same range and the same box you're expected to fit into. No nuance or context is considered, and there is no gender differentiation. And the blood test for TSH is the first and often the *only* test that most practitioners run to assess your thyroid.

Here's what that looks like in real life: A woman walks into her doctor's office with a TSH of 3.8 mIU/L. She's exhausted, gaining weight, can't focus, has zero libido, and is barely making it through the day without crying in her car. But she's "fine," her doctor says. No medication is offered. No deeper testing is pursued. There's just a generic reassurance that her TSH is "in range." Never mind that she feels like a shell of herself. Never mind that her body is screaming for help.

Meanwhile, another woman comes in with a TSH of 0.3 mIU/L. She's been taking prescription T4 and T3 for hypothyroidism and feeling better than she has in years. Her brain fog is gone, the weight is finally coming off, her energy is back, and she's sleeping like a human again. But instead of being able to celebrate her progress, she gets a call from her doctor saying she's overmedicated and needs to cut her dose immediately. What do you think is going to happen?

The system has failed these women. Neither one of them is being assessed in context. Their labs are being read like red lights and green lights, rather than as part of a full diagnostic picture. No one's asking how they feel. No one's looking at their free T3 or reverse T3 or even bothering to connect their symptoms to their broader hormonal function. Their providers are reacting to a single number.

Doctors aren't doing this to be cruel or deliberately neglectful. It's how they were trained. Most conventional physicians are taught to look for disease, not dysfunction. They feel that their purpose is to ensure that your life isn't at risk, not to make sure you feel good. And medical insurance doesn't pay for "feeling better"; it pays for diagnosing and treating International Classification of Diseases (IDC)–coded conditions. If you're not diagnosable by conventional criteria, your symptoms often go unsupported.

I want to tell you about Ava, who had seen six different doctors by the time she found me. She was forty-one, a working mom of two, and her labs kept coming back stamped with that same word: *normal*. Her TSH was 3.2 mIU/L (within "normal" limits). Her free T4 was midrange. Her doctor had told her, "You're doing great. Keep it up."

But Ava didn't feel great. She couldn't lose the fifteen pounds she had gained in less than a year. She always felt cold. Her skin was dry. Her hair was thinning. Her brain felt like cotton batting. One morning, she had left her laptop in the fridge and her yogurt in the car. Her health was going downhill, and no one had any answers beyond "Maybe try eating less."

When I ordered a full thyroid panel, which always includes free T3, reverse T3, and thyroid antibodies as well as TSH and T4, we found that her free T3 was completely tanked, her reverse T3 was sky-high, and her TPO antibodies were elevated. Textbook thyroid dysfunction. But none of her previous doctors had caught it because they never tested deeply enough, and they weren't looking at the results with Ava's well-being as the priority.

I also have patients whose stories are the flip side of Ava's. My patient Jenna had already found her groove: She was sleeping, she was clearheaded, her energy was back, and the weight had started to come off. Her thyroid medication included T3 and was working beautifully. But when she visited her endocrinologist, he panicked because her latest TSH was 0.2 mIU/L, below the accepted normal range of 0.4 to 4.5 mIU/L. "You're hyper," he said, meaning hyperthyroid. "This is dangerous. You need to cut your dose immediately."

Never mind that her free T3 was in the optimal range and her reverse T3 was low. On top of that, she felt better than she had in years. The doctor hadn't asked how she was doing or feeling; he had simply seen the number and pulled the alarm. Jenna listened to the doctor's advice, reduced her dosage, and within a few weeks was feeling foggy again. Her energy disappeared. The scale crept up. Her hair started falling out again. She was back to square one.

Which is why I'll say it again: The difference between "normal" and optimal matters. In functional medicine, we define optimal thyroid function based on the ranges in which people feel good. That can mean a TSH somewhere between 0.0 and 2.0 mIU/L, as long as your other numbers are in order. "Optimal" means that your free T3, the active, usable thyroid hormone, is sitting in the upper quarter of the lab range, not near the bottom. It means that your reverse T3 is low, your antibodies are calm, and your body is functioning like the well-oiled machine it was built to be.

Whenever I see women posting their numbers on my Facebook group page, almost every time, their labs show only TSH and maybe free T4. That's it. Because that's all their provider ordered.

This isn't on them. Even when women know something's wrong, they're fighting years of conditioning to trust whatever their doctor says. Most of us were raised to believe that doctors are the ultimate authority, that questioning them is dangerous, that if we speak up or push back, we're being difficult. For generations, women have been told to be quiet, be polite, and be grateful for whatever scraps of attention they're given in the exam room.

That's why I'm repeating myself, because I want this to really sink in. You cannot accept "normal" as the final answer when it comes to your labs. You need to have the full blood work panel done. You must push for real answers. You deserve not just normal but optimal results. Because the second you settle for anything less, you're giving your life over to someone else's idea of "good enough."

Let's look at the relevant lab tests and blood markers one by one, and I'll show you exactly what optimal looks like. It's my hope that the next time you get your results, you won't be confused, you'll feel confident, and you'll know what to ask. Most important, you'll know how to take back control.

The Thyroid Panel: Your Guide to the Tests You Need

I'll say it again and again: Too many doctors and other practitioners today refuse to run a full set of thyroid labs. They'll test for TSH or maybe T4 and stop there, but those tests alone fail to give a complete picture of what is going on with your thyroid. Even worse, they can point you in the wrong direction when it comes to treatment. If a provider hasn't run enough tests to have all the facts, dosing their patients with thyroid meds is like shooting in the dark.

At my clinic, we do a full panel of blood work on new patients every time, regardless of what they think they know about their thyroid or how many prior test results they show up with. This is because, as you hopefully know by now, none of these hormones can be looked at in isolation, and the HPT axis is vulnerable to many factors. You can't know what's happening with T3 by looking only at T4. You can't know if someone has Hashimoto's, or to what degree, without testing for antibodies. And you can't possibly prescribe someone the right replacement hormones without looking at their reverse T3 to see if their body is converting T4 properly.

So what tests do you need? A complete panel of thyroid labs should include tests for the following:

- Thyroid-stimulating hormone (TSH)
- Free T4
- Free T3
- Reverse T3
- Thyroid antibodies: TgAb and TPO

I'm going to unpack each of these tests so you know exactly what to look for and what your results mean—with the goal of them being not normal but *optimal*. And one more thing. If you remember nothing else, please remember this hard-and-fast rule: If your doctor won't run a full panel that includes tests for free T3, reverse T3, and both thyroid antibodies, it's time to get a new doctor.

TSH

First up is the conventional medicine favorite: the test for thyroid-stimulating hormone (TSH). It's the go-to test anytime you walk into a doctor's office and complain about weight gain, fatigue, depression, constipation, hair loss, or anything else that gives even a hint of thyroid problems. They'll test your TSH and send you on your merry way.

But TSH is not a thyroid hormone. I'll yell that louder for the people in the back: TSH IS NOT MADE BY YOUR THYROID! It's made by your pituitary gland, and its one job is to yell at your thyroid when it's being lazy. When the thyroid is sluggish and your body is falling apart, the pituitary gland is standing there screaming, "Hellooooo? You wanna wake up and do something today?"

You know when you've told your teenager five different times to clean his room? And to not leave his sweaty gym socks and crusty underwear in the bathroom? The first time, you're cool. Maybe even the second. But by round three or four, your voice starts to rise. By round five? You're basically unhinged.

That's exactly how your brain feels when your thyroid's slacking. Your pituitary starts yelling louder, and your TSH starts rising because the pituitary is pissed. It's trying to kick your thyroid into gear.

That's why TSH lab results are interpreted backward, because they're inversely related to your amount of thyroid hormone. TSH is one of the only markers where "high" means "low." If you have high TSH, your thyroid is underperforming. It's not producing enough of the indicated hormones, and your brain's trying to rally the troops. Your brain is essentially doing the same thing as when you yell at your kid repeatedly to clean his room.

What is "too high" or abnormal for TSH? Here's where it gets interesting: Decades ago, doctors considered a TSH of 10 mIU/L to be fine. Ten! That is your pituitary yelling *very* loudly. You could basically be comatose from low thyroid, and the medical folks would pat you on the head and say, "Everything looks great." Eventually, someone figured out that maybe that was a bad idea, and the upper limit dropped to 6 mIU/L—still way too high to feel like a normal human being. Then, years later, the upper limit dropped to 4.5 mIU/L and held there. That's better but, in my opinion, still not right.

In functional medicine, we pursue an optimal TSH level of under 2.0 mIU/L. In my experience, that's where people's energy starts coming back, the scale stops creeping up, their brain fog lifts, and they don't want to scream into a pillow every morning.

"But what if my TSH gets too low?" you ask. "Isn't that dangerous?"

Let's unpack one of the scare tactics you'll confront in thyroid care. Someone will tell you that low TSH means that you are hyperthyroid, the condition where you have *too much* thyroid hormone. Someone may tell you that low TSH will cause osteoporosis, too. Both statements are incorrect. If your doctor is inducing fear over a low TSH result and warning you that it will cause heart failure, bone loss, or something equally terrifying, you need a new doctor. That's not me being dramatic, that's me being honest.

A suppressed TSH level, when paired with proper treatment and stable free T3 and free T4 levels, is not dangerous. In fact, it's sometimes intentional. After a thyroid cancer diagnosis and thyroidectomy, patients are kept at a TSH of 0.0001 mIU/L on purpose to prevent thyroid tissue from growing back. That suppression is done under medical supervision for years, and no one is sounding the alarm about their bones crumbling. So why would a TSH of 0.3 mIU/L suddenly be labeled "too low" or "dangerous" in someone without cancer? It's not.

I've been on T3-only therapy for seventeen years. My TSH? 0.0007 mIU/L. I'm healthy, strong, and living proof that a suppressed TSH level can be completely safe when managed correctly. I'm still lifting weights, still running a business, still writing this book, still alive and thriving, and there's not a fracture in sight. In my practice, we don't panic over a low TSH level. We look at you and what you're taking for thyroid replacement, ask how you feel, and then look at your *other* thyroid lab values since the other values are more important. The blood markers for free T3, free T4, reverse T3, and those sneaky little antibodies tell us way more about your thyroid health than TSH ever can.

Myth buster: A low TSH by itself is not a problem. It's the *context* of your other labs and how you feel that tell the real story.

Key Takeaways: The Test for TSH

- TSH is not a thyroid hormone, it's a megaphone from your brain.
- High TSH = underperforming thyroid.
- Optimal TSH range: 0.5–2.0 mIU/L.
- TSH naturally drops when you're on proper thyroid treatment, especially T3.
- A low TSH level does *not* equal danger if the rest of your labs are okay.

Low TSH: What You've Been Told Versus the Reality

What You've Been Told	The Reality
Low TSH means you're hyperthyroid.	Nope. A single TSH number can't diagnose hyperthyroidism. You have to look at free T3, free T4, and how you actually feel.
Low TSH will cause osteoporosis.	Not automatically. Bone health is about nutrient status, hormone balance, and lifestyle. Suppressed TSH alone isn't the villain.
Low TSH will cause heart failure.	Only if your thyroid is completely unmanaged. With proper treatment and monitoring, your heart will be just fine.
Low TSH is always dangerous.	Wrong again. Sometimes we *want* it to be suppressed—such as after thyroid cancer—and people live for decades that way without a problem.

What About Hyperthyroidism?

Before we move on to other tests, I want to address the hyperthyroid question. A doctor may tell you that you're hyperthyroid based on nothing more than a suppressed TSH level. This is one of the most common misdiagnoses I see, especially in patients who are on thyroid medication and finally starting to feel human again. If your doctor is looking only at your TSH and ignoring your free T3, free T4, and how you feel, they're working with incomplete information.

Suppressed TSH *can* indicate hyperthyroidism. But let's put that into context so you know exactly where the line is. If you're on thyroid medication and your doctor is panicking over a low TSH, clutching their pearls, and tossing around the word *hyper*, it's time to take a deep breath and lean in to some common sense.

When someone is truly hyperthyroid, they know it. There is no guesswork, no subtlety, no "Hmm, maybe I feel a little off." You don't need a lab test to tell you that something is jacked. You're anxious. You're amped up. You're jittery, sweaty, icky, and sticky. Your heart is racing. You can't sleep. You feel like a shaken-up soda bottle with no cap. You are uncomfortable and wired. That, my friend, is what hyperthyroidism feels like.

In hyperthyroidism, in which your thyroid is overproducing hormones on its own, all three key markers fall into a specific pattern: Your TSH is low, and both your free T4 and free T3 are elevated, often well above the optimal range. *All three* must show those patterns *at the same time* for it to be true hyperthyroidism. And if you're overmedicated and starting to feel icky and sticky, those are the labs that will confirm it.

But—and this is important—we do not diagnose hyperthyroidism based on TSH testing alone. Ever. Why? Because of everything I talked about above. Once you're on thyroid medication, especially one that includes T3, your TSH can be suppressed and you can still feel perfectly normal, even amazing. If your doctor starts fretting about hyperthyroidism, insist on a full panel of thyroid labs to confirm it.

Free T4: The Inactive Hormone That Gets Too Much Attention

This is the second most common test that doctors run. But even TSH with a free T4 test is not a comprehensive thyroid panel. Running just those two is barely scratching the surface. I start giving Instagram "experts" the side-eye hard when they talk about optimal T4 levels.

T4 is your inactive thyroid hormone. You might recall my personal story from earlier in the book and how I thought a T4 prescription was going to change my life. I didn't know then what you know now: That little pill was simply replacing inactive thyroid hormone. It still had to be converted into T3, the form your body uses. T4 is the couch potato of thyroid hormones. It's just hanging out, waiting for its moment to be turned into something useful.

When we test free T4, we're looking at the unbound, "active-in-waiting" version of that hormone. It's not doing much yet, but it's available. Blood work that measures free T4 reflects both what your thyroid is naturally pumping out (if you still have your thyroid gland) and any synthetic T4 supplied by medication you're taking (such as levothyroxine or Synthroid). Therefore blood tests for T4 measure internal production and external input combined. The standard "normal" range for free T4 is 0.8 to 1.8 ng/dL (nanograms per deciliter, which is the way that US labs measure the amount of hormone in a specific volume of blood).

You might see some functional practitioners say that the sweet spot for free T4 is 1.5 ng/dL. That sounds logical, maybe. It's the middle of the normal range, right? But here's the problem: T4 must convert to T3 for your body to use it, and T4 has *two* paths it can go down. It can convert to free T3, the hero hormone that makes you energetic, sharp, lean, and alive, or it can go down the dark alley and become reverse T3, the anti-thyroid hormone that shuts everything down and pushes your body into hibernation mode.

When I see a free T4 level above 1.3 ng/dL, I start placing bets in my head about how jacked up the reverse T3 is going to be. Because here's what I know after working with thousands of patients: If you have too much T4 in your system, from either natural production or synthetics, your body reads it as an excess of energy potential, i.e., too much T3. To protect itself from going hyperthyroid, it slams on the brakes and starts converting T4 to reverse T3 instead of the active form (T3) you need. Reverse T3 blocks all the active T3 you have, which is why you are stuck feeling like crap with all the symptoms of hypothyroidism even though your labs look "good."

In my world, we don't chase T4 levels. We never say, "Let's add more T4 meds to get that number up"—because more T4 doesn't always mean more energy, weight loss, or brainpower. In fact, it can trigger the opposite.

In my experience, the true optimal range for free T4 is less than 1.3 ng/dL. That's right, lower than what most "experts" are telling you. And if you're like me and your thyroid doesn't convert worth a damn? You can have a rock-bottom free T4 and still feel fantastic if your T3 is dialed in. My free T4 level is 0.2 ng/dL, basically nonexistent, because I'm on T3-only therapy and have been for seventeen years. My reverse T3 is also low, and that's okay. That's my body, and that's *my* unique chemistry.

In a perfect world, I'd love to take both T4 and T3. Having both hormones on board is ideal for many people because it mimics what is naturally produced by a healthy thyroid. But my body doesn't want or need T4. I've tried it, and every time, my reverse T3 climbed, my symptoms came back, and I felt worse. For me, low free T4 is not a problem; it's what works.

This is why I will never put thyroid treatment into a one-size-fits-all box. The thyroid is nuanced. Every patient is unique. What works beautifully for one person can backfire for another. Effective thyroid care considers the whole picture—your labs, your symptoms, your history, and how you feel—and adjusts treatment to fit you, not a chart or a formula. My numbers might not look "classically optimal" on paper, but they're optimal for me, and that's the only thing that matters.

My advice is to have a little T4, but if it makes things worse for you, don't obsess over it. This is one test where the numbers when you're optimized might look very different from someone else's and still be perfect for you.

It's worth noting that there is also a blood test that measures your total T4—that is, your free T4 and bound T4 together. But it is considered to be less accurate and in my opinion is not worth doing. The only number you really need is the one that tells you how much active, unbound, and readily available T4 you have circulating in your bloodstream at any given time.

Key Takeaways: The Test for Free T4
- T4 is inactive. It needs to be converted to T3 to be useful.
- Too much T4 may result in high reverse T3, which means you're feeling like trash.
- Don't chase a 1.5 ng/dL level just because someone on Instagram said it's the magic number.
- Ideally, free T4 is less than 1.3 ng/dL, maybe even lower, depending on your conversion capability.
- If you have a "normal" T4 level and still feel crappy, get tested for reverse T3. That may very well tell the true story.

Free T3: The Hormone That Gives You Life
Now we get to the real MVP, my favorite lab marker, the hormone that has the ability to change your life: free T3. The blood tests for free T3 and reverse T3 are the only ones that truly indicate what's happening with your thyroid gland. Having these tests ordered by your clinician should be nonnegotiable every time you get your thyroid checked.

In my opinion, as stated in the hard-and-fast rule above that you *must* live by, if your doctor says no to testing free T3 and reverse T3, it's time to get a new doctor. No excuses, no debate. These lab tests cost your provider nothing. Ordering all of them takes no extra time. If doctors aren't ordering them, it's likely because they have no idea what the results measure or what they indicate for thyroid care. Either way, an uncooperative and uninformed clinician has no business managing your thyroid.

When we measure free T3, we're looking at the active, unbound thyroid hormone. Remember, "unbound" means it's not attached to TBG carrier proteins in your blood, so it is free to enter your cells and do its job. Bound hormone is like money that's tied up in a long-term investment; it exists, but you can't use it right now. Free T3 is like cash in your hand, ready to spend. It's the hormone your body uses, the one that does the work.

When it comes to free T3, as I said previously, we're not aiming for "normal." Normal lab ranges are based on statistical averages of the population, which often means the bare minimum you need to avoid disease. Translation: *You're technically alive, so congratulations, you're not dead yet.* But alive and thriving are two very different things.

We want optimal. In my experience, optimal for free T3 means being in the upper quadrant, the top 25 percent of the lab range. This is where most people see their energy return, weight stabilize, brain fog lift, mood improve, hair grow back, and digestion normalize. Free T3 is measured in pg/mL (picograms per milliliter) and the "normal" range for adults is 2.0 to 4.4 pg/mL. This means that the optimal range is roughly 3.5 to 4.4 pg/mL, or even a little higher if that's where you feel amazing and your symptoms are gone. I believe that when it comes to free T3, it's okay to be slightly above range as long as you are not experiencing any symptoms of hyperthyroidism. If you are feeling jittery or anxious and your free T3 is above range, it's time to look deeper into hyperthyroidism. But if you're above range and feel incredible, keep rolling with that elevated free T3. It's all about personalization!

Here's the best part: The unit of measurement does not matter when you're using the quadrant method. Whether your lab uses pg/mL, pmol/L (as they do in Europe), or something else, all you have to do is take the range printed on your lab report, divide it into four equal parts, and aim for that top quarter, or even slightly above if that's where you feel your best.

A note about getting accurate results: If you're on any kind of prescription T3, such as liothyronine or Cytomel, compounded meds, or even a thyroid glandular like Armour Thyroid or NP Thyroid, it's essential that you withhold your dose for eighteen to twenty-four hours before being tested for free T3. Here's why: After you take T3, it peaks in your blood at about four hours, then starts to drop. This is why we often prescribe T3 in two daily doses, to keep its level steady. In contrast, T4 is like a tortoise: slow, steady, and fine to take once a day. T3 is like a hare—fast in and out.

If you test at the peak, four hours after taking your morning T3, your free T3 will look high, and not just a little high, but flagged way above the lab's "normal" range. (If you do not spike high at the peak, that is a massive red flag, because it means you are severely undermedicated. But in most cases, you will see that peak number soar.) Here's the danger: If the person reading your labs does not understand thyroid physiology— and let's be honest, that includes most practitioners—they will assume that you are overmedicated. The "solution" in their mind? Cut your T3 dose. And because you were not overmedicated to begin with, you are going to drop back into hypothyroidism. The fatigue will hit, the weight will come back, your hair will fall out, your brain will fog over, and all the progress you made will vanish.

Even practitioners who claim to know about thyroid care can get this wrong. Why? Because there is no such thing as an optimal reference range for peak T3 in functional medicine. It does not exist. This is because everyone's optimal dose is—and should be—different. Here's what this looks like.

- I'm prescribed 75 mcg of T3 twice a day. If I test at the peak, my free T3 is 16 pg/mL.
- One of my patients takes 25 mcg twice a day. Her peak is 6 pg/mL.
- Another patient takes 40 mcg twice a day. His peak is 10 pg/mL.

Who is "in range"? Does my 16 pg/mL mean that I'm overmedicated? Absolutely not. If you drop my T3 dose based on that number, I will gain ten pounds in a week and slide into clinical depression. I know because I have experimented with lowering my dose, and that was exactly what happened.

Now imagine thyroid patients everywhere being told that their T3 is "too high" because they were accidentally tested at its peak. Every one of them will end up hypothyroid again, all because of improper testing.

Testing T3 between eighteen and twenty-four hours after your last dose is the only way to get a number that truly reflects your baseline. Anything else is guesswork, and guesswork ruins lives.

Key Takeaways: The Test for Free T3

- Free T3 is the active thyroid hormone, the one that matters.
- You want your free T3 level to be in the upper quadrant of the lab range, or higher if that's where you feel great.
- Always be tested eighteen to twenty-four hours after your last T3 dose.
- Testing at the peak (three to four hours postdose) tells you nothing. Avoid doing so.

Reverse T3: Your Metabolism's Emergency Brake

This lab marker tells us more than most doctors give it credit for. Yet it's one of the most dismissed and ignored tests in conventional medicine. I sometimes call reverse T3 the anti-thyroid hormone because it often works against us. It can be the reason you're still tired, gaining weight, and wondering what the hell is wrong even though your labs are "normal."

Reverse T3 is built into your biology as a survival mechanism, and we do need it. It has the ability to determine whether your metabolism is chugging along as usual or if it's slamming on the brakes. If you're ever in a traumatic accident, if you're lying in an ICU bed postsurgery, if you're battling a life-threatening infection, you want your reverse T3 to go up. Your body activates an enzyme that converts T4 to reverse T3, which blocks the activity of free T3 to slow your metabolism way down. Doing so helps your body conserve energy so that all its resources can be redirected to healing. It's your body saying, "Hey, now is not the time to burn through body fat, regrow your hair, or balance your checkbook. Now is the time to survive."

But what if your body thinks it's in survival mode when in reality you're just trying to live your life? You're trying to work, raise kids, socialize, run a business, go to the gym, juggle a million things. And instead of supporting you in that, your body slams on the brakes. It thinks you're dying, when you're just trying to meet a deadline. That's reverse T3 gone rogue. And that's when it becomes a problem.

Remember that T4 is what converts to reverse T3. If you have high levels of T4 either from your thyroid pumping it out or because you're taking a higher dose of T4 medication than you need, your body will switch to converting it to reverse T3. It's meant as a check on excess T3, but this switch happens regardless of whether your body has more T3 than it needs. Reverse T3 climbs and blocks whatever T3 is already there. Hypothyroidism sets in, and soon your metabolism is stuck, your brain is foggy, and you struggle to get out of bed in the morning.

But T4 overload isn't the only culprit. As we've said, converting T4 to T3 is hard work for your body. And a lot of factors can interfere with that process and push conversion toward reverse T3 instead of free T3. I talked about this in chapter 1, but here's a lovely little laundry list of just some of the things that can drive up your reverse T3.[2]

- Insulin resistance (93 percent of Americans have it)
- Low progesterone or estrogen dominance
- High or low cortisol
- Low iodine
- Low selenium
- Low magnesium
- Low vitamin A
- Low vitamin D
- Low ferritin (iron stores)
- Viral infections
- Chronic stress
- Genetic SNPs that impair conversion

SNP, pronounced "snip," is short for "single-nucleotide polymor-phism." That's just science-speak for a tiny variation in your DNA, one "letter" in your genetic code that's different from what's typical. It may seem small, but some of these variations can change the way your body works, including how efficiently you convert T4 to T3. If you have a SNP that slows down this conversion pathway, it doesn't matter how much T4 you have, you'll still struggle to get enough active T3, and you'll feel all the low-thyroid symptoms that come with it.

Reverse T3 is measured in ng/dL (nanograms per deciliter), and the "normal" range is considered to be 8 to 25 ng/dL. In my world, based on my own experience and that of thousands of my patients, the optimal range for reverse T3 is less than 12 ng/dL. That's the number. Less than 12. If your test gives you a different range, simply cut the range in half and aim to stay under that number.

Key Takeaways: The Test for Reverse T3
- Reverse T3 is your body's emergency brake, built for trauma, not for everyday life.
- Reverse T3 rises when T4 is too high or when T4 to T3 conversion is blocked.
- Causes of elevated reverse T3 include T4 overload, nutrient deficiencies, insulin resistance, stress, low sex hormones, and more.
- Elevated reverse T3 guarantees symptoms—no exceptions.
- Optimal range: less than 12 ng/dL in the United States.
- You must treat reverse T3 seriously and adjust your plan accordingly.

Thyroid Antibodies: TPO Antibodies and TgAb
As we've said, Hashimoto's thyroiditis is the autoimmune form of hypo-thyroidism, where your immune system mistakes your thyroid gland for the enemy. Hashimoto's is not something to be scared of, but it is some-thing you want to understand. Because when you know exactly what is

happening in your body, you can take the right course of action and take back control of your health.

There are two tests that matter when it comes to diagnosing Hashimoto's: thyroid peroxidase (TPO) antibodies and thyroglobulin antibodies (TgAb). These are both immune system markers, and before you ask, you absolutely want to get tested for both. Please do not let your doctor test just one. I see this happen all the time. Patients come in having had only their TPO antibodies tested, the test comes back negative, and they think they're in the clear. Meanwhile, their TgAb is lit up like a Christmas tree.

Let's talk about TgAb first, because it doesn't get enough love. Thyroglobulin is a protein made only by the thyroid gland. It is stored inside the thyroid follicles and acts as a building block and storage unit for your thyroid hormones, T4 and T3. Under normal, healthy circumstances, thyroglobulin stays inside the thyroid. It doesn't wander into the bloodstream.

But when your thyroid is under autoimmune attack from Hashimoto's, it becomes damaged and inflamed. Thyroglobulin leaks into the bloodstream, your immune system sees it, panics, and sends thyroglobulin antibodies to go after it. So when TgAb shows up in labs, that tells us there's an autoimmune response under way. The soldiers are out, and the thyroid is under fire.

TgAb is measured in IU/mL (international units per milliliter). The reference range will vary depending on the lab. Many US labs consider anything less than 1 IU/mL as negative, while others view 0 to 4 IU/mL as normal.

Here's the problem. With the "less than 1" standard, you might not even see a number unless you're clearly above 1 IU/mL. With a 0 to 4 IU/mL range, you could be at 1, 2, or 3 IU/mL and still be labeled normal. Your doctor may tell you that you do not have Hashimoto's. That is why TgAb can be trickier to interpret and why it's so important to test for both TgAb and TPO antibodies to get the full picture.

The fact is, any antibody is an antibody. Any antibody is a soldier. Here's the part you will hear me say again and again until every doctor on the planet gets it: *Any* presence of TgAb signals that there is an autoimmune response happening. I don't care if your lab says that the reference range is under 9, under 34, or under 1 IU/mL. If your lab shows any number above zero, you have antibodies. You have Hashimoto's.

TgAb is just one piece of the puzzle, but it's a powerful one. Now we'll deal with TPO antibodies.

TPO stands for thyroid peroxidase, an enzyme that sits on the outer surface of thyroid cells and plays a crucial role in producing thyroid hormones. When you have antibodies against the TPO enzyme, your immune system is interfering directly with hormone production. This is why TPO antibodies are often the first test ordered, and why they are positive in more than 90 percent of people with Hashimoto's.

TPO antibodies are also measured in IU/mL, and just like TgAb, the reference range depends on the lab. Some use less than 9 IU/mL as normal, others less than 34 IU/mL. But again, the goal is zero. *Any* TPO antibody is a soldier attacking your thyroid, and even a small number is a sign that your immune system is in the fight.

You don't need both antibodies to be elevated to have Hashimoto's. One is enough. And you can have Hashimoto's with no antibodies showing up at all. This is called seronegative Hashimoto's, and it's real. Studies show that 5 to 10 percent of Hashimoto's patients test negative for both antibodies.[3] This is why we also look at your full thyroid panel—TSH, free T3, free T4, and reverse T3—and, of course, your symptoms.

You could also be doing so many things right that your antibodies have dropped to zero: eating gluten free, living an anti-inflammatory lifestyle, taking the right supplements. That doesn't mean you never had Hashimoto's. It means you are managing it like a pro.

Bottom line: If you have ever had positive TPO antibodies or TgAb, you have Hashimoto's thyroiditis. If your mom, sister, aunt, or grandma has it and you have symptoms, you probably have it, too. If you have an-other autoimmune condition and hypothyroid symptoms, chances are high that Hashimoto's is in the picture. Autoimmune conditions tend to cluster. Where there is one, there are often more.

The Stages of Hashimoto's Disease: How the Labs Look

Hashimoto's doesn't go from zero to sixty overnight. It unfolds in stages, and the testing for both antibodies and thyroid hormones can look different at each stage. However, each stage is also an opportunity to step in and intervene. Here's what you can expect.

Stage 1: Genetic Predisposition

You've got the genes. Maybe you have other autoimmune conditions. Your labs look okay. Your TSH is normal, your free T3 and free T4 are solid. You may have antibodies, but you have no symptoms.

This is the time to act. Start taking black cumin seed oil supplements. Go gluten free. Reduce stress. Support your immune system. You might be able to keep it at bay forever.

Stage 2: Subclinical Hypothyroidism

In stage 2, your TSH might start climbing. You now have antibodies. Free T3 and T4 might be shifting just a bit. Maybe you have a few symptoms: mild fatigue, unexplained weight gain, feeling cold. You might even still be asymptomatic.

But this is your thyroid getting tired. It's soldiering on, still showing up to work even while it's getting punched in the face. This is your critical window to jump in and take action.

Stage 3: Full-Blown Hypothyroidism

Your symptoms are loud. You have fatigue, weight gain, depression, hair loss, dry skin, constipation, the whole deal. Your antibodies are elevated. Your TSH is high. Your T3 and T4 are in the toilet. Your thyroid is no longer producing hormones the way it should.

This is when conventional medical practitioners finally pay attention. This is when they say, "Oh, look, Susie, your TSH is above 4.5. Let's give you some Synthroid." But if you're not being treated properly—and by properly, I do not mean T4-only—you are never going to be optimized. You're always going to suffer symptoms on T4 only. Always. Synthroid alone is not enough. You need T3 as well.

Stage 4: Advanced Destruction

Chronic symptoms, nodules, a shrinking thyroid gland. Maybe your antibodies even start to go down, not because you're getting better, but because your thyroid is almost gone. There's nothing left for your antibodies to attack.

Stage 5: End-Stage Hashimoto's

Your thyroid gland is basically gone. Your hypothyroid symptoms persist. Your TSH is high, your free T3 and free T4 are low. Your antibodies might be low or undetectable, not because you're healed but because there's nothing left to destroy.

You'll need lifelong thyroid hormone replacement, but that's okay. With proper treatment (and again, *not* T4 only), you can still live a fully optimized life.

Can You Go into Remission?

Remission from Hashimoto's is possible, and antibodies can return to zero. It can take time, sometimes years, but it's possible. You'll find more guidance on this in part III, but here are some things you can do to counter your body's autoimmune activity.

- Go gluten free (gliadin, the key protein found in wheat, looks almost identical to thyroglobulin, which spurs further attacks).

- Take vitamin D3 (10,000 IU daily).

- Take selenium (100 mcg/day, not 200).

- Take zinc.

- Take iodine (start low and slow).

- Take black cumin seed oil, one of the most powerful anti-inflammatory, anti-autoimmune supplements.

- Manage your stress.

- Get plenty of sleep.

- Avoid processed junk food.

You don't have to go on an extensive autoimmune protocol unless you're in a flare-up. You don't have to lose your mind over food. Just be smart, consistent, and targeted. Hashimoto's is manageable and treatable. But it starts with *knowing*. And now you do.

Now What? You Have the Labs. You Have the Truth. Let's Go!

So now you have your lab results in front of you. You've decoded them. You've circled what's outside the optimal range. And now you're sitting there thinking, "Holy shit. Years ago, when I started gaining weight, when I told my doctor I was exhausted, when I was begging for help, they brushed me off. And now I can see it right here in black and white. It *was* thyroid. It was always thyroid."

What do you do now?

I'm going to walk you through it, because this next part gets nuanced. You absolutely need to be working with a thyroid expert who knows what they're doing, but I also want to give you the power to go into your next appointment with confidence, clarity, and the ability to steer the conversation. You're no longer a confused patient. You're the one holding the map.

In chapter 7, I'll tell you exactly how to talk to your doctor to progress the conversation and get the help you need. For now, I'm going to show you how to figure out your next steps using your test results.

We're going on a choose-your-own thyroid adventure!

Step 1: Look at Your TSH

The reference range for TSH is standardized across labs at about 0.4 to 4.5 mIU/L. The optimal level in functional medicine is under 2.0 mIU/L.

If your TSH is above 2.0 mIU/L and you have three or more of the top symptoms of hypothyroidism (or if you crushed the thyroid self-assessment at the beginning of this book), congratulations, you've got thyroid dysfunction. Let's unpack where to go next.

Step 2: Look at Your Free T4

The reference range for free T4 can vary slightly by lab but is usually 0.8 to 1.8 ng/dL. The optimal level of free T4 is less than 1.3 ng/dL.

If you're not on thyroid medication and your free T4 is above 1.5 ng/dL, yet you're tired, bloated, brain fogged, and gaining weight, that tells me you're not converting thyroid hormone properly. Your body might be making T4, but it is not turning it into usable T3.

If your free T4 is above 1.5 ng/dL, immediately look at your reverse T3.

Step 3: Look at Your Reverse T3

The typical lab range for reverse T3 is 8 to 25 ng/dL. The optimal level is under 12 ng/dL.

If your reverse T3 is greater than 12 ng/dL, you have conversion problems. Something has caused your body to stop converting T4 to T3, and you're getting reverse T3 instead. A heightened level of reverse T3 may be pushing your body into human dormancy mode. At the very least, you feel like crap.

At this point, you know that a prescription is needed, because you need to replace the T3 your body isn't making. See Step 4. In this scenario, I would prescribe more T3 medication than T4, or possibly even T3 only.

Step 4: Adjust the T3/T4 Ratio Based on Your Reverse T3 Level

When prescribing replacement thyroid hormones, it's important to get the exact proportions of T3 to T4 correct. Often, you want a little bit of

T4, but if your body truly can't convert it, you'll only be adding fuel to the reverse T3 dumpster fire. In those cases, it is better to prescribe T3 only. How do we know if your body can handle T4? We look at your reverse T3 number to provide the answer.

Reverse T3 Between 12 and 16 ng/dL

You can still have a little T4 on board, but we skew the ratio heavily in favor of T3. Think 80 to 90 percent T3, 10 to 20 percent T4.

We'd start Mary on 5 mcg of T3 twice daily and increase the dosage slowly. Her T4 dosage would be kept low at 25 mcg twice daily or maybe 50 mcg once daily. We'd retest in four to six weeks to ensure that her reverse T3 is coming down and her free T3 is climbing into the optimal range.

Reverse T3 Between 16 and 24 ng/dL

We use the same strategy, but we go even lighter on the T4. T4 is the only hormone that converts to reverse T3, so if your body is doing a poor job of converting it properly, we don't want to keep dumping in more.

I'd put Mary on a lower 12.5 mcg dose of T4 twice daily but start with the same 5 mcg of T3 twice daily, and then increase T3 as needed.

Reverse T3 Flagged as High (>24 ng/dL)

You need T3 only. Period. At these levels, your reverse T3 is like a roadblock for your metabolism. We are not going to add any more T4 into that equation. Your body needs help, not more confusion. You can start with 5 mcg of T3 twice daily and go up as needed until symptoms disappear.

In all scenarios, make sure you do your best to ascertain *why* your reverse T3 is high—for example, due to nutrient deficiency or insulin resistance—and take steps to fix the root while you tweak the meds.

Reverse T3 Level	Treatment Approach	Example Starting Point
12–16 ng/dL	80–90% T3, 10–20% T4	T3: 5 mcg twice daily; T4: 25–50 mcg daily
16–24 ng/dL	Go lighter on T4; start low-dose T3 and build	T3: 5 mcg twice daily; T4: 12.5 mcg daily
>24 ng/dL	T3 only; remove all T4	T3 only, dosing based on symptoms

Step 5: Look at Your Free T3

The typical range for free T3 is 2.0 to 4.4 pg/mL. Optimal is the top 25 percent of the range, roughly 3.5 to 4.4 pg/mL.

If your reverse T3 is fine (under 12 ng/dL) but your free T3 is nowhere near the top quarter of the range *and* you have symptoms, that is also an indication that you are not converting well and need more active thyroid hormone. Since reverse T3 is low, we know that at least some of your T4 is converting into usable T3, but we still add prescription T3 to make sure you are getting enough.

In this scenario you have some options: You can opt for natural desiccated thyroid, such as Armour Thyroid, REN Thyroid, or NP Thyroid, which contain both T4 and T3, or you can take synthetic T4/T3 combo therapy with separate dosing. For example, you could start with 25 to 100 mcg of T4 and add T3 gradually until you land at your optimal dose. I'll talk more about medications in the next chapter.

• • •

Congratulations! You're not in the dark anymore. You know your numbers. You know what they mean. You know where you should be. And now you know what to do about it. You are not going for "normal," you are going for optimal, and that's a game changer. To learn how medications can support you in your quest, read on.

Chapter 6

The Right Prescription: Optimizing Medication

Dr. Amie, what's your favorite thyroid medication for getting some-one optimized?" I get this question all the time, and my answer never changes: The best thyroid medication is the one that works for *you* in the combination that works for *you* and at the dosage that works for *you*. Because when it comes to the thyroid, there is no one-size-fits-all plan. Getting someone optimized is always a nuanced process.

The thyroid protocol taught in medical school is basic and straight-forward: Test the patient's TSH, and if it's over 4.5 mIU/L, prescribe T4 replacement medication. That's it. No discussion of free T3, no digging into the exact reasons for symptoms, no adjusting based on how the pa-tient feels.

Here's how that looks in real life: A woman comes into the doctor's office, dragging herself through the door. Her hair is breaking off, and she has brain fog so thick she forgot where she parked. She tells the doc-tor that she's exhausted and gaining weight despite barely eating, she can't sleep, and her mood is in the gutter.

Doctor: Let's run your labs . . . Well, Sally, your TSH is 5.1 mIU/L. That means you have hypothyroidism. Let me write you a prescription for levothyroxine, 25 micrograms. Here you go.
Sally: Thank you. So will we retest soon to make sure it's working?
Doctor: Yes, in six months.

Sally: But what if I need an increase or a different medication?

Doctor: Nope, we'll retest you in six months. See you then!

That's the standard approach. You get a prescription, a pat on the back, and a promise to check your TSH again in six months. No real monitoring. No conversation about whether your body is converting T4 to active T3. No plan for what happens if you're still symptomatic. And it is so far from useful that I can hardly put it into words.

Clinicians who are instructors at the American Academy of Anti-Aging Medicine (A4M), a global organization devoted to longevity and regenerative medicine, teach a simple but powerful truth: T4-only therapy works for a small minority of patients with hypothyroidism. In their clinical experience, only about 2 percent of people feel fully optimized on T4 alone. The other 98 percent need a combination of T4 plus T3 to have a real shot at feeling like themselves again. They believe strongly that thyroid treatment must be multifaceted and tailored to each patient if it is going to work.

In my decades of practice, I have seen this to be true. Two percent of patients may feel fully optimized while taking T4, but they are not the people who show up at our clinic. I can confidently say that 100 percent of the patients we see in my practice—and we have seen thousands— require some form of T3, either T3 only or a combination therapy of T3 plus T4, because that's what it takes to feel the benefits of medication, and that's what it takes to get optimized.

In the conventional medicine world, however, combination therapy is used much less frequently. A 2017 survey of US endocrinologists found that only 18 percent would even attempt a T4/T3 combination in patients who still had symptoms despite having a "normal" TSH.[1] That means that over 80 percent of endocrinologists will keep you on T4 alone, no matter how miserable you are feeling.

It remains a mystery why doctors do not learn more about the thyroid gland in medical school. A national survey of US endocrinology fellows found that endocrinology exposure during medical school was sparse, with only 2.8 percent reporting their school even had an endocrinology student interest group and nearly 60 percent saying their exposure to endocrinology in the curriculum was inadequate.[2] Add to this the reality that fewer doctors are pursuing endocrinology specialties, and we can begin to understand why thyroid-related care is difficult to come by. Most medical students get only a brief mention of thyroid disorders in their broad internal medicine lectures, and any hands-on thyroid training takes place during residency and fellowships. Physicians who have already chosen other specialties by that point never get that deeper thyroid education. In my opinion, the thyroid does not get the respect it deserves in the standard med school curriculum, given its outsized role in our overall health. Big Pharma also has a growing influence on what gets prioritized in medical school training, which is worth thinking about.

If you want to roll the dice and bet your future health on every word your conventional doctor says, go ahead. But you would have better odds gambling in Vegas. Thyroid care is one area where I strongly believe it is essential to take a broader approach and work with a provider who will be flexible and proactive—and that starts with utilizing available medications.

Thyroid Medication—Thyroid Hormone Replacement

When I recommend thyroid medication, I don't mean quickly giving out prescriptions to cover up symptoms. I'm talking about thyroid hormone replacement, which means replacing what your body can't produce or convert properly. Prescriptions for antidepressants, sleeping pills, and blood pressure medications are Band-Aid treatments that, while they might quiet a symptom or two, leave the underlying problem unaddressed and continuing to do damage.

Thyroid hormone replacement is different. It's not about masking how you feel; it's about giving your body the hormone it needs to function at every level, from your metabolism to mood and your ability to get through a day without crashing. When it is properly prescribed, monitored, and adjusted, thyroid medication gives you back your life because it actually restores what's missing.

Consider Lisa. When she came to me, she was taking three medications: one for anxiety, one for insomnia, and one for high blood pressure. Her lab results showed a sluggish thyroid that wasn't being addressed. Once we replaced her missing T3 and optimized her hormone levels, her anxiety melted away, she slept through the night, her blood pressure normalized, and all three Band-Aid prescriptions were gone. That's the power of fixing the real problem.

When your thyroid hormones are low or not converting, your cells are starving. They don't have the fuel they need to power your metabolism, brain, digestion, and energy. Replacement is not a shortcut or a crutch, it is a necessity. It is no different from replacing insulin in someone with type 1 diabetes. No medical practitioner would ever look at a diabetic and say, "Let's see if you can heal naturally first. Maybe you don't really need insulin." That would be reckless and dangerous. Yet I see so many women who feel guilty or ashamed about needing thyroid hormone replacement, as if it means they've failed or given up. That mindset only keeps you stuck.

So let me be crystal clear: Thyroid hormone replacement is not excessive or unnecessary. It is a real, evidence-based treatment that supports every single cell in your body. If your body can't make thyroid hormone, you need to replace it to survive. When you start seeing it this way, it stops feeling like just taking another pill and starts feeling like what it is: giving your body what it desperately needs to function because it can no longer make these vital hormones on its own.

If you've been hesitant to take thyroid medication because you are worried that it is somehow "unnatural," know this: You are not taking something foreign or toxic. Yes, the medications are made by pharmaceutical companies, but they are all *bioidentical* hormones—that is, hormones that are chemically identical in their molecular structure to the ones your body produces naturally. The term *bioidentical* comes up often in the context of menopause and hormone replacement therapy (HRT), when we talk about replacing lost estradiol and progesterone with synthetic, chemically identical versions to alleviate the symptoms of menopause. HRT is widely accepted as the first-choice treatment for menopause and with good reason. The same thinking applies here: Biosynthetic T4 levothyroxine and biosynthetic T3 liothyronine are molecularly identical to the hormones your own thyroid makes. Whether they come in a standard commercial form or a compounded capsule, they can work incredibly well to get you optimized as long as dosing and conversion are correctly addressed.

Let's break down the different types of thyroid medication, because understanding the various names, forms, and sources will give you the power to choose what works for you.

Natural Desiccated Thyroid (NDT)

Natural desiccated thyroid (NDT) medication is derived from the dried thyroid glands of pigs and contains both T4 and T3 in fixed ratios, along with other thyroid hormones naturally found in the gland. For many patients, NDT has been a breakthrough. It was, in fact, the very first pharmacological treatment for hypothyroidism, developed in the late nineteenth century.

But I want to clear something up right now: NDT isn't "natural" in the way some people define that term, although it does have a biological source. It is also produced by pharmaceutical companies, but instead of being manufactured like synthetic T4 and T3, its bioactive ingredient comes from the dried thyroid gland of pigs.

Why pigs? As it happens, the porcine thyroid hormone ratio is almost identical to that of humans—about 80 percent T4 and 20 percent T3. That T3 content is one reason many patients feel better on NDT, as opposed to taking T4 alone. For many, making the switch from T4-only medication to NDT is beneficial.

Although it has been used for over a century and has the word *natural* on the label, NDT is not a perfect fit for everyone. Like every other medication, it comes with pros and cons. One of the drawbacks is that NDT is still mostly T4. Remember that T4 can also convert to reverse T3, your body's brake pedal. If your body is a poor converter to T3 and most of your medication is T4, you may not feel much better at all. You might even feel worse. If all that T4 is driving up your reverse T3, you do not get a gold star for choosing something "natural."

Overall, NDT is well tolerated, and the 20 percent T3 it contains is often described as a gentler form of T3. People who are hypersensitive to stimulants or medications sometimes do better on NDT, provided that their bodies convert the T4 portion effectively.

The big-name brands of NDT are Armour Thyroid, REN Thyroid, and NP Thyroid. I have seen patients thrive on Armour Thyroid but feel awful on NP Thyroid, as well as the opposite. Even with NDT, getting to the combination of supports that works for you and your biochemistry is a nuanced process, so I urge you to be patient with this part. The formulas are similar, but the fillers, inactive ingredients, and even sourcing of each medication can differ, and these factors can affect how each one works for you and your thyroid gland. You can see why working with someone who truly understands thyroid treatment is so important—because sometimes the difference between feeling terrible and feeling great comes down to something as simple as switching brands.

There is some potential for NDT to trigger an autoimmune flare. Now let me clarify: This is my theory based on what I've seen in my practice. This is not backed by published research because current clinical data on NDT focus on symptoms, quality of life, and metabolic side effects, not immune activation. So as with any great debate, I'm going to lay out my argument and I'll let you decide if it applies to you.

Since roughly 95 percent of hypothyroidism is Hashimoto's, your immune system likely already views your thyroid as the enemy and is sending antibodies to attack it. Because NDT is made from pig thyroid, your immune system may recognize it as similar (but not identical) to your own thyroid tissue, prompting your antibodies to launch another attack. This doesn't happen to everyone, but when it does, every dose can feel like a fresh battle inside your body. But please listen . . . if NDT is working for you, don't panic when you read this. Just pay attention, and if you notice your symptoms creeping back in or you feel worse over time, reassess, retest, and maybe try a different combination of thyroid hormone.

When it comes to any medication or treatment, the real questions are always: Are you getting better? Are your symptoms improving? If you are taking something and you still feel terrible, your body is telling you that it is time for a change. Doing the same thing over a longer period likely won't get you a different result.

In my clinic, if NDT works for you, we use it. If adding a little extra T3 makes it even better, we do that, too. You don't necessarily have to choose one or the other. Sometimes a combination of treatments does the best job.

The War over NDT

At the time of this writing, there is a storm brewing over access to NDT. On August 6, 2025, the Food and Drug Administration (FDA) posted an industry advisory alerting all manufacturers, importers, and distributors of NDT that it intends to take action against these products, labeling them as unapproved animal-derived thyroid products. The FDA acknowledges that NDT has been in use for over a century yet claims that it has not been adequately assessed for safety and effectiveness.

Its stated concerns are inconsistent potency, potential viral contamination due to the animal source, and the presence of what it calls "supraphysiological levels" of T3 that, in its opinion, could lead to hyperthyroidism. The FDA also notes that NDT is no longer the predominant form of thyroid hormone replacement, pointing to the FDA-approved synthetics T3 liothyronine, approved in 1956, and T4 levothyroxine, approved in 2002, as preferred options. Interestingly, T3 was approved decades before T4, yet T4-only therapy has become far more common in conventional practice.

At this point, we do not know what will happen. Petitions are circulating to stop the FDA from pulling NDT. And if I can share my personal opinion, it is absolutely ridiculous, ludicrous, and mind-blowing that an agency devoted to the health and well-being of Americans would tell the estimated 1.5 million patients currently taking NDT that they can no longer have the one medication that works for them. Many of these patients have already tried T4-only therapy and failed to get relief, had adverse reactions, or simply did not tolerate it.

If you have read this far in the book, you already know how hard it is to get optimized, first convincing your doctor to test, then to treat you properly, then to prescribe enough T3 to get you feeling like yourself again. Now imagine finally finding the medication that gets you there—only to have to fight for the right to keep taking it.

The Biosynthetic Options: T4 and T3 Medications

Synthetic replacements for human thyroid hormone have been in use since the 1950s. Both T4 and T3 can be created in a laboratory using a multistep process of chemical synthesis, starting with the amino acid tyrosine. The process ultimately produces medications that are structurally identical to the hormones made by the human body. Synthetic thyroid hormones are a safe and effective long-term treatment for hypothyroidism and when prescribed correctly can be nothing less than life changing. You will get maximum benefit from these medications by working with a provider who believes in personalization.

Synthetic T4

Synthetic T4, known by the generic name levothyroxine (brand names include Synthroid, Levoxyl, and Unithroid), is made by multiple manufacturers. Even though the active ingredient is the same, the fillers, binders, and manufacturing processes can vary. Those variations can make a difference in how you feel.

Some patients do great for years on one specific generic, and when their pharmacy switches its preferred manufacturer without warning, their symptoms return within weeks. There they are again: fatigue, brain fog, and weight gain, and they are baffled as to why. If you find a generic version that works well for you, write down the manufacturer's name and keep it somewhere safe. Request that your pharmacy order that exact one for you every time. If it can't, find a pharmacy that will. Your thyroid is too important to leave to chance.

Sometimes the difference is not just the manufacturer, it's the generic medication itself. Many contain fillers such as lactose, dyes, or trace amounts of gluten. For some people, especially those with celiac disease or gluten sensitivity, that's enough to stall progress. In these cases, switching from generic levothyroxine to brand-name Synthroid can make a noticeable difference.

A step up from Synthroid is Tirosint. Tirosint is a soft gel capsule that contains only levothyroxine, glycerin, gelatin, and water, with no dyes, lactose, or gluten and few excipients. Because it's so clean, most people tolerate it extremely well. The downside is that it's more expensive, and most insurance companies require you to fail both generic levothyroxine and Synthroid before they will cover it.

Above Tirosint is Tirosint-SOL, which comes in a liquid capsule or liquid solution. This form contains zero fillers, making it the purest T4 option available. It's ideal for patients with sensitivities, absorption issues, or severe autoimmune reactions to fillers. The drawback is cost. Tirosint-SOL is rarely covered by insurance and can be pricey.

As I've said, the amount of T4 you need depends on how well your body converts T4 to T3 and what your reverse T3 level looks like. Some people can tolerate higher amounts of T4, while others need only a small dose paired with their T3 to feel their best.

Synthetic T3

T3 is the active form of thyroid hormone, the one your cells actually use. If you've read the earlier chapters, you know that your body is supposed to convert T4 to T3, but many people are poor converters. They have plenty of T4 floating around, but very little of it is making the leap to become T3, leaving them symptomatic despite having "normal" labs.

This is where synthetic T3 comes in. If you have conversion issues, adding T3 to your thyroid regimen can ensure that your active T3 levels are consistently where they need to be to keep you optimized and feeling like yourself.

T3 comes in various strengths in the United States: 5, 25, and 50 mcg tablets are the most common. This means that you have a lot of options for dosing and that you can find the exact amount of T3 that works for you. Most of the time, we start small with the 5 mcg pills and slowly build up until you're taking around 25 mcg once or twice a day. At that point, we can usually switch you to the 25 mcg tablet so you're not juggling a handful of pills.

One thing you need to know: T3 acts fast, but it doesn't hang around in your system very long. When we talk about the half-life of a medication, we're talking about how long it takes for the medication to drop to half its strength in your body. T3 has a much shorter half-life—approximately twenty-four hours—than T4 does. Because it moves through your system so quickly, it's usually best to split your T3 dose. Taking it twice a day helps keep your levels steady and prevents the big peaks and crashes that can happen if you take it all at once.

The generic name for T3 is liothyronine (brand name Cytomel). Just as with T4, different manufacturers put in different fillers and ingredients, and those little changes can make a big difference in how you feel. Once you find a version that works for you, stick with it. Brand consistency matters more than most people realize.

Here's a quick story on that topic. One day I picked up my T3 refill and noticed that the pills looked smaller. I called the pharmacy to confirm that it was still the right dose. The person there said yes but told me that the pharmacy had switched suppliers due to supply chain issues. Within a week on the new pills, I noticed that I was feeling anxious. That's not typical for me. I retraced my steps, wondering what had changed. Then I remembered the new T3 manufacturer. I called the pharmacy and asked it to order the version I had been taking before. It did, and almost immediately everything shifted back. My anxiety disappeared, and I felt like myself again. That experience was a powerful reminder of how much small details can matter. The fillers, the sourcing, even the manufacturer can all impact how you feel. This is why personalization matters so much in thyroid treatment.

In my experience, generic T3 works well and has few fillers. Most of my patients do not need to switch to the brand Cytomel, which saves them money because even if you're fortunate enough to have medical insurance, insurers rarely want to cover brand-name treatments.

When You Need T3 Only

Combining T4 with T3 or adding T3 to NDT works well most of the time, but there is a small group of patients who need T3 alone. There aren't any statistics on how many people fall into this group, but I would estimate that it's 1 to 2 percent at most. In my practice over the last twenty years, out of thousands of patients, I have had maybe twenty-five who were truly T3 only. That shows you just how rare this really is. But when someone needs T3 only, they need T3 only.

I know this because, as I mentioned earlier, I am a T3-only person. You can find out if you are only through trial and error. If we're working together to optimize you, and after incrementally lowering your T4 prescription because your symptoms aren't improving and your reverse T3 is staying high, I'll suspect that you might be a nonconverter. At that point, we'll pull the T4 out entirely, shift to T3 only, and see what happens.

When we are tweaking medication regimens, I always remind my patients to pay close attention to their body. Be aware of small changes. A competent thyroid expert will ask you often if your symptoms have improved since T4 was removed.

Do you feel better? Good.

If you stay on T3 only until you feel stable and your symptoms don't change from day to day, it can be possible to add in a little T4 again in a couple of months. We start very small. And you pay close attention to your body.

Did nothing change? Good.

Did your symptoms stay away? Perfect.

Did fatigue creep back in? Are you feeling sluggish, retaining water, or getting that old brain fog again? If that happens and stays consistent, we pull the T4 back out.

Again, do you feel better?

If the answer is yes, we might wait a month or two and try one more time. If we add T4 twice and the same thing happens both times, you can be confident that you are T3 only.

I did this experiment on my own body. Every time I tried to add even

25 mcg of T4, I would gain ten pounds in a week and feel what I now know was clinical depression. It happened so quickly that my reverse T3 didn't even have time to spike. Even that little dose of T4 sent my body straight into hypothyroid mode. Later, I completed genetic testing, and sure enough, I have a SNP on my DIO1 and DIO2 genes, which means that I have about a 50 percent chance of being a nonconverter.[3] And in this case, the genes were right. My body cannot convert T4.

When I talk about real T3-only patients, I often reference my patient Amanda. Before she came to me, she had seen a functional doctor who had an arbitrary cap in his mind about how much T3 any patient should have, which was no more than 20 mcg daily. Then she went to a thyroid expert who would prescribe only natural desiccated thyroid medication, which contains both T3 and T4.

When I reviewed Amanda's long history of labs and saw consistently elevated reverse T3, it was clear that she should be a T3-only person. Once we removed the T4 and put her on T3 alone, everything changed. Her strength came back. Her muscles came back. She lost the excess fat. Her brain fog lifted. Every symptom she had been battling for years finally started to fade, and within a couple of months, she got her life back.

All this happened after years of being on T4 that had done nothing but drive her reverse T3 higher and keep her stuck in hibernation mode.

It turned out that Amanda needed 50 mcg of T3 twice a day to feel healthy. So much for her first doctor's 20 mcg limit. And while NDT does contain 20 percent T3, Amanda's body needed 100 percent T3. The NDT approach didn't work for her, either.

The free T3 optimization table below is your quick reference tool for understanding where your free T3 levels fall, what that means for your thyroid function, and how your treatment might be adjusted. While lab reports will give you a "normal" range, you now know from reading chapter 5 that *optimal* is very different. This chart tells you whether you're underdosed, sitting in a "normal but not optimal" zone, right in the sweet spot, or possibly too high. It also offers next-step considerations based on both your numbers and your symptoms—because the right dose is never determined by lab results alone; it's a combination of labs, how you feel, and how your body responds over time.

Free T3 Level	What It Means	Treatment Approach/Next Step
<2.0 pg/mL	Well below normal, significant hypothyroid symptoms likely	Increase T3 dose; evaluate conversion issues and root causes.
2.0–3.4 pg/mL	Within normal range but not optimal	Add or adjust T3 to push into top 25% of range.
3.5–4.4 pg/mL	Optimal range (top 25% of lab range)	Maintain current therapy; continue root cause support.
>4.4 pg/mL	Possible overmedication or poor cellular uptake, or it can be optimal for some individuals to be above the upper limit	Reevaluate dose; look for factors blocking T3 at the cell level; or leave dose alone and enjoy optimized living.

Compounded Thyroid Medications

Compounded thyroid medications are the ultimate examples of nuanced, patient-specific thyroid care, because they are custom-made by a pharmacy to match your exact needs. Instead of handing you the standard tablets from a big manufacturer, a compounding pharmacy makes your medication to order. It might contain T4, T3, or a combination of both in precise ratios, doses, and forms—such as slow-release T3—that are not available in standard commercial formulations. Compounded forms can be particularly helpful for patients who cannot tolerate fillers, dyes, or certain inactive ingredients in manufactured drugs.

Compounding is especially relevant in the case of T3. Remember, T4 is the tortoise and T3 is the hare. T3 jumps into action quickly, it starts working almost right away, it peaks at around four hours, and then it tapers off. That's why we usually dose it twice a day, whereas T4 is slow and steady enough to take once daily.

But here's the catch: Some people just don't tolerate T3 at full speed. They might feel jittery, overstimulated, or as though their heart is racing. For those people, a compounded slow-release version of T3 can be a lifesaver. Instead of flooding the system all at once, the compounded formula is designed to release T3 more gradually, stretching out the peak and smoothing the effect across the day. Think of it as putting the hare on a leash—it's still fast, still effective, but controlled.

There's a belief floating around that "compounded" automatically means "better." It feels pure, closer to nature, safer somehow. I get it, I used to think that, too. But here's the truth: In my twenty-five years of practice, I have never once seen a patient fully optimized on compounded thyroid medication. Not once. I wish I had a clear explanation for why. Maybe it is the source of the raw thyroid hormone. Maybe it is the way the pharmacy prepares it. I honestly cannot say. What I do know is this: Every patient who has walked into my office who was on compounded thyroid medication was still hypothyroid. And not just a little hypothyroid but deeply hypothyroid, even the ones who were supposedly on higher doses of T3. It is almost as if their body was absorbing only half of what was written on the bottle.

Now, I love compounding pharmacies. We use them all the time for bioidentical hormones and peptides. They are excellent in those areas. But when it comes to thyroid replacement, I turn to compounded meds in only two specific situations. The first, as I mentioned above, is in the case of patients who are so hypersensitive to T3 that the regular tablets make them feel jittery or overstimulated. In those cases, a compounded slow-release version can make a huge difference, because it trickles into the body gradually instead of hitting all at once. The second is in the case of patients with celiac disease, who need 100 percent assurance that their medication is gluten free.

For everyone else? Standard thyroid medications usually work far better. But here is what happens: Someone reads a blog post or sees a Facebook comment claiming that Synthroid has gluten in it or that liothyronine contains corn, and suddenly they are terrified. They call the office asking to be switched to a compounded medication because they are worried about fillers.

I try to explain it this way: Walking through the bakery at your grocery store gives you more gluten exposure than your thyroid pill does. You inhale more gluten and corn in that one walk than you will ever get from the tiny amount of stabilizer in your medication. Just recently, I had a call with a woman who was panicked about a speck of corn-derived maltodextrin in her prescription. I told her, "If that is your biggest fear, then you can never eat out at a restaurant again, *ever*, and you can never walk past a bakery again for the rest of your life. Because the exposure from cross-contamination, cooking methods, and even inhalation will be far greater than the trace amount in that pill."

While compounding has its place, please believe me when I say that it is not the magic answer for thyroid treatment. If anything, it often keeps women stuck, chasing "pure" medication while their symptoms continue.

All thyroid medications can technically be compounded, and sometimes this is exactly what sensitive patients need. That said, most people do perfectly fine with the standard tablets, so compounding usually isn't necessary unless you have side effects or react to fillers.

What If You Don't Have a Thyroid?

If your thyroid has been removed, partially taken out, ablated, or destroyed with radioactive iodine, this section is for you. Whether the decision was based on cancer, nodules, Graves' disease, or a well-meaning doctor who told you it was your best option, the reality is that now your thyroid isn't doing what it was intended to. And your entire body feels it.

As you know by now, your thyroid gland produced two essential hormones, T3 and T4, when it was inside your body and functioning properly. But it didn't just create them; it also played a central role in converting T4 to T3. Unfortunately, too many patients are handed a prescription for T4 only after their thyroid is taken out or destroyed. That's like removing the engine from your car and expecting it to run because you filled the tank with gas.

The reality is that you are now fully dependent on outside hormones to replace what your body can no longer make *and* do. If you're being given only T4, you're addressing only half the problem. And in my opinion, treating a thyroidectomy patient with T4 only is medical malpractice.

This is where so many patients fall through the cracks. They go into surgery thinking that everything will be fine. One little pill, and they'll be back to normal. But instead, they start gaining weight, losing energy, feeling flat, anxious, foggy, inflamed. They show up to appointments desperate for answers and are told that everything looks fine. Their TSH is normal. Their T4 is normal. The doctor pats them on the back and sends them on their way. No one is looking at their free T3 or checking their reverse T3—as usual. But if your thyroid is gone, you are now dependent on medication to keep your entire system running. Your medication has to be dialed in with precision, and it has to include the hormone your body truly needs: T3.

For those of you who've had a partial thyroidectomy and were told that you didn't need medication, but ever since the surgery you've been feeling tired, gaining weight, or just not feeling right, this applies to you, too. Half a thyroid is still a compromised thyroid. It may not be enough to keep up with your body's demands, especially during stress or hormone shifts.

The answer is not to settle. The answer is not to stay on T4 and hope your body will magically figure it out. The answer is a comprehensive treatment plan that mimics what your thyroid used to do. That means T4 *and* T3, monitored and adjusted over time based on your labs and how you feel.

You can absolutely feel like yourself again after thyroid removal. But it starts with getting the right medication in the right form at the right dose.

• • •

I know that was a ton of information to digest, so I'll briefly summarize everything I covered above. Remember, knowledge is power!

Key Takeaways: Thyroid Medication

- There is no such thing as a single perfect thyroid medication. What works beautifully for one person may fail for another.
- T4 alone often does not get people optimized, and combining T4 and T3 in the right ratio can be life-changing.
- There are different forms of T4—generics and the brands Synthroid, Tirosint, and Tirosint-SOL—so a change in prescription or manufacturer can throw your body off.
- T3 is fast acting and usually needs to be dosed twice a day.
- A person can be sensitive to changes in source, dosage, and frequency.
- Natural desiccated thyroid (NDT) helps some people feel amazing, but it can be the wrong fit for others, especially for poor T4 converters with persistent reverse T3 issues.
- In rare cases, a patient needs to be T3 only, and trial and error is the only way to figure this out.
- Compounded medication can be helpful for those who are hypersensitive to T3 or who have celiac disease and must avoid any trace of gluten. But compounded thyroid medication is *not* a guaranteed better option in general.
- Thyroid medication done well is a nuanced and personalized process. It involves both you and your provider paying close attention to your symptoms and your body's responses, tracking your labs, and being willing to make adjustments until you feel your best.

Always remember: You have options. You are allowed to question, to ask, to test, and to try again. You do not have to accept feeling half alive. You deserve to feel vibrant, clear, and strong.

I believe that medication is your greatest ally, so bookmark this chapter and come back to it anytime you feel confused or overwhelmed. Use it to remind yourself that you are not stuck. Medication regimens can and should be tweaked and adjusted through *informed* trial and error until you feel like yourself again. You have every right to find exactly what works for you.

The Most Common Thyroid Medications

Medication	Type	Generic or Brand Name	Filler Content	Cost and Insurance	Key Advantages	Possible Drawbacks
Generic levothyroxine	T4	Multiple manufacturers	Varies; may contain dyes, lactose, or gluten	Usually cheapest, widely covered by insurance	Affordable; easy to access	Manufacturer changes can cause symptom flare-ups; fillers may trigger sensitivities.
Synthroid	T4	Brand name only	Fewer fillers than most generics	More expensive than generics; usually covered by insurance if generics fail	Consistent formulation; widely available	May still contain dyes and/or lactose; not as clean as Tirosint.
Tirosint	T4	Brand name only	Very few fillers; no dyes, lactose, or gluten	Higher cost; often requires prior authorization after generic medications and Synthroid fail	Highly tolerated; good for patients with sensitivities	There may be cost and insurance hurdles.
Tirosint-SOL	T4	Brand name only	No fillers	Most expensive; rarely covered by insurance	Purest T4 form; ideal for patients with severe sensitivities or absorption issues	Cost is high; insurance coverage is limited.
Generic liothyronine	T3	Multiple manufacturers	Very few fillers	Affordable; often covered by insurance	Fast acting; effective for poor converters	Manufacturer changes can affect tolerance; requires twice-daily dosing.
Cytomel	T3	Brand name only	Consistent formulation	Expensive; rarely covered by insurance	Consistent; some people prefer brand stability	Cost is high; there is no major advantage for most patients over generic versions.
Compounded slow-release T3	T3	Custom compounded	No standard fillers; tailored to patients	Not covered by insurance; cost varies	Ideal for hypersensitive patients; slow release	Requires access to a compounding pharmacy; cost is high; is not always necessary.
Compounded T4/T3 combination	T4 + T3	Custom compounded	No standard fillers; tailored to patient	Not covered by insurance; cost varies	Personalized ratio; filler free	May not perform better than separate dosing; may not be available.

Chapter 7

Navigating the Medical Maze: How to Find a Doctor

Your symptoms are gifts. Yes, I said it. And I mean all of them. They are gifts from your body that tell you something's off. Symptoms are your alert system, the signal that something needs your attention. They are the warning lights on the dashboard of your body, trying to get your attention before things break down entirely.

Sure, it doesn't feel like Christmas morning when your jeans won't button and you're so tired that you can barely get out of bed, let alone go to the gym. But our bodies weren't built to be fat, foggy, and fatigued. When those symptoms show up, you'd better believe there's a reason.

The beautiful part? When you pay attention to the signs and do the work to find the source, those symptoms can be reversed. That's why I call them gifts—even if they feel more like a flaming bag of poo on your doorstep.

So don't look a gift symptom in the mouth. Don't ignore the signs and put off addressing them until "one day" in some hypothetical future when you have more time. That day will never come; you know that. We must pay attention to the whispers from our body when they are still only whispers, because if we don't, they turn into screams.

The difference between me and every other "thyroid influencer" out there is that I don't pretend that a detox smoothie or essential oil will magically solve a medical condition. I know the power of thyroid hormone replacement. I know the life-changing effects of bioidentical hormone therapy. I will never lie to you and say you can heal your body "naturally" with a wand and a vision board. That's bullshit.

Sometimes you need actual medical intervention. Period. And this means you will need to seek out a doctor or another type of clinician with the right experience who can help you.

So where to start?

The Familiar Path: Conventional Medicine

Most people start with their primary care physician (if they have one) because that is who is supposed to care. Your family doctor is supposed to know you, and they should want to figure out what's going on. That's their job.

Unfortunately, most family doctors don't know much about the thyroid. They often know even less about hormones and women's health in general. They follow the textbook standard of care that we have already talked about: Test TSH, and if it is above 4.5 mIU/L, prescribe T4 medication. That's it. That is the protocol, and it is mediocre at best.

I am not saying that every primary care physician is clueless. You may find one with an open mind, and if you look hard, you might even find one who has been trained in how thyroid hormones work. But the vast majority do not understand the nuances of thyroid care—and as we've seen, nuances can make all the difference.

So maybe you think, "Okay, my ob-gyn deals with female stuff, they know about hormones, so they will get it." You would think that ob-gyns, of all people, would care about hormones, right? After all, one of their jobs is to help women get pregnant, stay pregnant, and deliver healthy babies. Estrogen, progesterone, and testosterone are all important in pregnancy, but so are thyroid hormones. You need thyroid hormones to conceive, to maintain a pregnancy, and to build a baby's brain properly.

Yet even though ob-gyns see hormone-related conditions such as polycystic ovary syndrome and endometriosis every day, most will still tell you that thyroid hormones are not worth testing. I can't tell you how many times I have heard, "My ob-gyn told me that hormones don't matter." I'm sorry . . . I beg your pardon? Your entire job involves hormones! And you are saying they do not matter?

After all this, you might think that endocrinologists would be the heroes in this story. After all, the word *endocrine*, which refers to the glands in your body that produce hormones, is right there in the name. Hormones and their associated glands are supposed to be the endocrinologist's specialty.

But I'm going to burst that bubble. I have been in this field for nearly thirty years and worked with patients in nine different countries. For years, I kept a list titled "Good Endocrinologists." It was a running list of the rare unicorns in conventional medicine who got it. Want to know how many names made it onto that list? Three. Three names in three decades across nine countries.

It is one of the most significant scams in modern medicine, the way endocrinology is practiced in the conventional system. Endocrinologists are supposed to be the experts in hormones, yet the vast majority stick to outdated, one-size-fits-all protocols that leave patients suffering. It's like the worst as-seen-on-TV product ever. Even a ShamWow works better than the average endocrinology appointment does.

My honest, best recommendation to you is: Don't expect an endocrinologist to save you. Save your time. Save your money. Save your sanity. Don't even bother. I know that's a hard truth to hear. And maybe some society of endocrinologists or medical organization is going to come after me. But I don't care. I promised I'd always keep it real with you. And this is me doing just that. I care much more about your life and health than I do about sparing someone's professional ego.

Here's the part that really breaks my heart: After bouncing from doctor to doctor, being dismissed and gaslit, most women are so relieved to finally get a diagnosis that they'll accept any treatment plan handed to them, no questions asked. They're exhausted, and they're desperate. So when the prescription pad comes out and they're given a T4-only med such as Synthroid or levothyroxine, they think, "Finally, this is it. I'm going to feel like myself again." I thought the same thing the first time I was given Synthroid. I wanted to believe *so badly* that the pill was going to fix me.

But that's where the next letdown begins.

T4 only doesn't work. You've heard me repeatedly on this. Even though docs are still being taught across the board in medical schools and continuing education that a T4-only prescription protocol is the gold standard, it simply does not work. Let me say it again: T4 only will not make you feel better.

But people don't know what they don't know. The truth is that most women who say, "I'm doing okay on T4" aren't aware of how bad they feel—until they feel better. They assume that the way they're feeling is "normal" because the doctors keep telling them their labs are fine. And if their labs are "normal," the medication must be working, right?

I'll never forget a conversation I had with a woman I sat next to on a flight. She was polished, professional, probably in her early forties. We struck up a casual airplane chat. She asked what I do, and I told her that I specialized in thyroid and hormone dysfunction. She lit up and said, "Oh! I have a thyroid issue." So naturally, I asked what she was taking. She told me that she was on Synthroid and "doing okay."

But when we got deeper into the conversation, she started telling me about how she was tired all the time, her clothes were fitting tighter, and she just didn't have the mental clarity she'd used to. She chalked it all up to aging. She didn't know any different. She thought she was doing "okay" because she had no idea what feeling good felt like anymore.

Always remember that "okay" is not the goal. Thriving is the goal. Waking up with energy, a sharp mind, a steady mood, a body that works for you and not against you—that is the goal. If you're on T4 and wondering why you still feel as though you're trudging through molasses, this is your moment. You're not going crazy, and you're not just getting older; you're just on the wrong treatment. You need a new provider—and it's time to fix that.

The Conventional Medicine Route: What to Ask Prospective Practitioners

If you are committed to staying in the world of conventional medicine, at least for now, there are ways you can vet prospective practitioners before you waste your time and money. You're not just looking for a doctor; you're looking for someone who understands how the thyroid works and how to treat it properly.

A lot of well-meaning guides out there will tell you to just "ask your local compounding pharmacy for a referral." You can try this, and you might even get a few names and phone numbers of "progressive" providers, but don't assume that they are any better equipped to treat you than the average conventional PCP. You can still find yourself sitting across from a doc who thinks T3 is dangerous or that testosterone is only for men.

Fortunately, because of this book, you are in the driver's seat and no longer going in blind. Your job is to interview and size up any new provider, whether they're a nurse practitioner or the new ob-gyn down the street, before you waste another minute of your life or another dollar from your bank account.

Before you make an appointment, pick up the phone and call the office. You are not being "difficult," you are not being "demanding." You are shopping for someone to manage your hormone health, and you have every right to ask questions and vet your doctor as you would a nanny, a housekeeper, a contractor, or a brain surgeon.

Ask the receptionist these questions:

- Does the provider routinely test for free T3 and reverse T3?
    - → The only acceptable answer here is yes.
- Does the provider currently treat patients with natural desiccated thyroid like Armour Thyroid or NP Thyroid?
    - → If they say no, that's a sign that they are probably not open-minded when it comes to thyroid care.

- Does the provider prescribe T3 medications such as liothyronine or Cytomel?
    - → If they say no, that's a deal breaker, and you should end the call.
- Does the provider have an upper dosing limit for T3 or Armour Thyroid that they refuse to exceed?
    - → The only acceptable answer here is "No, we do not have an upper limit; we dose T3 according to your needs."
- Does the provider use compounding pharmacies? If so, which ones?
    - → If they say no, that's not a good sign, because how will you get a compounded hormone medication if you need one?
- How long are appointments?
    - → A first appointment at my clinic is sixty minutes. Ten minutes or even twenty to thirty minutes is really not enough time for your provider to get a comprehensive health history.
- How do patients communicate with the provider between visits?
    - → It's important to have ongoing, open communication with your provider when you are tweaking and calibrating thyroid medications. If you experience unusual symptoms or side effects, you want someone who will respond quickly. No "We'll see you in six months."

The Other Path: Functional Medicine

At this point, you might be feeling discouraged because I just shot down all the obvious options for how to get help. Don't worry; I promise that I'm going to tell you how to get help and what to look for when you do.

I am a functional medicine provider. My entire team practices functional medicine. I studied it. I use it. I respect it. Functional medicine, at its core, is about getting to the root cause of health problems and diseases instead of slapping on another Band-Aid prescription and calling it a day. It looks at the whole body. It acknowledges that sometimes medication is the answer, but it also recognizes that lifestyle, nutrition, gut health, and hormone balance matter just as much.

Functional medicine can be an excellent option for thyroid care if, and only if, you know how to navigate that world. At its best, functional medicine is beautiful, powerful, everything that Western medicine has forgotten how to be. But lately, "functional" has become nothing more than a marketing word, so this path has potential pitfalls of its own.

Functional medicine used to be a sacred space. It attracted the rebel doctors, the thinkers, the problem solvers, the ones who were sick of insurance companies dictating what care should look like, so they decided to break out and do things differently. But then came the money. Insurance didn't cover functional medicine or integrative care, so patients paid out of pocket. Other doctors started to take notice. What did some of them do? They took a weekend course, slapped "functional medicine" onto their website, and started charging cash as though they'd just cracked the code for longevity. But they hadn't really learned anything. And they're still operating from a conventional mindset: T4-only prescriptions, fear of T3, refusal to touch testosterone or other hormones, and the same tired dosing limits they learned in medical school. They give you the exact same care you'd get by walking into your PCP's office with a $10 co-pay, only now they're charging you hundreds of dollars.

I've had patients come to me who have spent thousands, even *tens* of thousands, of dollars on so-called functional doctors who had the title, a pretty website, and a Zen office aesthetic. But when they showed me the labs those doctors had ordered, they were seriously lacking: no free T3, no reverse T3, no antibodies. That right there tells me that someone has no clue what they're doing when it comes to thyroid.

There are also true functional medicine providers who have the credentials and education, who have been through extensive multiyear programs such as the ones at the Institute for Functional Medicine or Functional Medicine University, so on paper they look fantastic. But when you check their website, they claim to do it all: autoimmune disease, fertility, mold, Lyme disease, small intestine bacterial overgrowth (SIBO), menopause, gut health, hormones, weight loss, men's health, detox, genetics, mindset, metabolism, and oh, yes—thyroid. You name it, they treat it. It's like flipping through a functional medicine Cheesecake Factory menu.

Conventional medicine has specialties for a reason, so why should functional medicine be any different? I'm not knocking these doctors' training, but let's be honest—how in the hell can you specialize in everything? You can't. Not in medicine, not in life, and definitely not in thyroid care. These practitioners try to be jacks-of-all-trades but are masters of none. If you go to a gut specialist or a Lyme disease specialist, why would you expect them to understand the nuances of thyroid function? It doesn't make sense.

At my clinic, we specialize in thyroid and hormone balancing. We call ourselves "functional" because we look at the whole body and we understand that the thyroid doesn't operate in isolation. We consider the gut, adrenals, insulin, estrogen dominance, all of it. But we're clear: We are thyroid and hormone experts. That's our lane. And if we hit a wall where deeper expertise is needed—for example, if we believe there's a cardiovascular issue or your lipid panel looks wonky—we will refer you to someone else. Because we're not going to bullshit our patients, take their money, and leave them sicker and more confused than when they came in.

If seeking help from conventional medical providers has cost you co-pays, time, and precious months of your life feeling like garbage, at least you haven't dropped tens of thousands of dollars on that disappointment. The functional medicine marketing machine can wreck your wallet fast. I'd say the average woman who goes down the functional medicine rabbit hole ends up spending somewhere between five and ten thousand dollars on everything from specialty supplements to provider-branded detoxes before she realizes that the missing piece is working with someone who specializes in the thyroid and understands hormone replacement therapy—down to the nitty-gritty, cellular-level details.

So be aware: When it comes to functional medicine, you don't need a provider who knows a little bit about everything. You need one who knows *your* problem—thyroid—inside and out. That's when the healing begins.

The Functional Medicine Route: What to Ask Prospective Practitioners

Just because someone uses the word *functional* or *integrative* in their bio doesn't mean they have a clue as to how to treat your thyroid. Even if you think you've found a reputable functional practitioner, you should absolutely still use all the vetting questions I listed earlier, plus a few more.

With integrative medicine, it should be a given that someone is going to look at your sex hormones alongside your thyroid. Real functional care looks at everything together, because your thyroid and your sex hormones are a tag team, and you can't treat one and ghost the other. This is critical to untangling the mess of symptoms that is thyropause. If you are a woman over the age of forty with thyroid problems, chances are that perimenopause and menopause are in the mix, too. And I hate to break it to you, but if your doctor treats one and not the other, you won't get better. You can't fully return to being happy and healthy unless your sex hormones—estradiol, testosterone, and progesterone—are taken into account and optimized right along with your T3 and T4.

It would be great if we could also rely on conventional doctors to test for sex hormones and consider the interplay between perimenopause and your thyroid, but the conventional doctor who does so is more than a unicorn—they're one in a billion. But functional medicine is another story. You have a right to expect that any functional thyroid expert worth their creds (and their price tag) will test for sex hormones and treat you as necessary to correct any imbalances and restore you to full hormone health.

Here's what to ask when vetting a functional or integrative practitioner, whether you are speaking to a receptionist or the doctor:

- Do they prescribe T3 regularly? (Not "Can they?" but "Do they?")
- Do they prescribe a variety of thyroid medications—synthetic, natural desiccated thyroid, and compounded—or do they prescribe only NDT?

- Will they individualize your dosing—or do they stick to one-size-fits-all protocols?
  - → Every aspect of hormone and thyroid treatment should be customized to your needs, your labs, your symptoms, your response. No two people require the exact same protocol, because no two people have the same biology. With functional practitioners, you need to make sure they walk the walk and don't just pay lip service to a "personalized experience."
- Do they have a cap for dosing T3?
- Do they monitor reverse T3 at every visit?
- Do they believe that sex hormones and thyroid function are connected?
- Do they address sex hormones alongside thyroid treatment? Will they run tests for those?
  - → Labs for sex hormones should include your levels of: the three estrogens (estradiol, estrone, and estriol), progesterone, free and total testosterone, sex hormone–binding globulin (SHBG), dihydroepiandrosterone (DHEA), and dihydrotestosterone (DHT).
- Do they treat thyroid and sex hormones together?
- Do they offer a full range of delivery options for sex hormones based on individual needs, including oral pills, creams, troches, patches, and injectables?
  - → If they prescribe only hormone pellets, that's a business model, not a treatment plan. You're not here to be locked into some cookie-cutter "care package" that doesn't care.
- What will the length of the first visit be?
- What are their communication channels like, and can I message the provider directly?

This is your script. Walk in with it, own it, and never let anyone make you feel as though you're asking for too much. You're not. You're asking for the care you deserve. And if they can't offer it? Move on. There are providers who can and will. You *can* find someone who will help you. But if you shortchange the vetting process, pick the clinic down the street because it's easy to get to, or fall for the shiny branding without asking the hard questions, don't be shocked when you're still fat, foggy, and fatigued—and ten grand poorer.

When you do this right, when you ask the hard questions and hold the line, that's when things will start to change.

Beware! Pop-Up Telehealth Clinics Are Not the Answer

Unless you've been living under a rock or are somehow immune to Facebook ads, you've probably seen the flashy new wave of online hormone clinics. They promise to fix your fatigue, melt your belly fat, and hand you prescriptions with just a few clicks and a friendly Zoom call with a mystery provider. Sounds convenient, right? A little *too* convenient. While I fully appreciate telehealth and it has its time and place, these cookie-cutter, one-size-fits-all operations that are springing up on every corner are the ones you need to watch out for.

Here's what usually happens: You fill out an online form. You check a few boxes. You maybe upload a selfie. And then, within twenty-four hours, there's a prescription on the way, written by some faceless, rotating "provider" you've never met and will never see again.

Oh, and there are no labs. Or maybe minimal labs—if you're lucky. Often these clinics don't test at all because testing takes time, and they are in the business of speed, not personalization. Meanwhile, they're handing out testosterone like candy, putting every man on the same dose and every woman on the same protocol, usually too high and almost always wrong. I've even heard of T3 being prescribed without any real monitoring. They're treating humans like algorithms. And you are a living, breathing, beautifully complex human being whose body deserves to be treated with nuance, precision, and above all, respect.

We had a patient go all the way through our program, do five months of work, and achieve full optimization and beautiful thyroid and hormone balance. She felt amazing. Then she decided to "cut costs" and jumped ship to one of those pop-up hormone clinics that advertised cheaper follow-ups and flat-fee hormone replacement. And what happened? It offered only one delivery method for each hormone: cream testosterone, cream estrogen, and oral progesterone. No personalization or adjustments were available, and there was definitely no nuance. She crashed—hard. She came back to our clinic six months later feeling like a shell of her former self. We had to rebuild her thyroid health from scratch. Her "money-saving" move cost her double and set her health back by half a year.

So here's my word of warning: You don't save money by going cheap on your thyroid medications, you save money by skipping the crap that doesn't work. Cut costs in other areas, but please don't skimp on your health! Use GoodRx to save money on prescriptions. Cut back on supplements. I would rather you take four good supplements than twenty half-assed ones and waste your money.

Your hormones give you life, vitality, metabolism, great hair, a good mood, a healthy libido, and joy. They are not optional. They are not replaceable. They are not where you should be bargain hunting.

How to Talk to Your Doctor To Get What You Need

Now that you've figured out where to go (or at least ruled out where not to go), it's time for the next hurdle: opening your mouth and not freezing like a deer in headlights once you're finally sitting in front of the doctor you hope will help you.

You've done the work. You've learned the labs. You know the lies. Now it's time to step up to the plate and use that knowledge to get the care you deserve.

The first rule of thyroid club? Walk in with a plan. And here's how you do it.

1. Present Your Symptom List

I don't care whether you're walking into a conventional clinic or a functional practice or having a Zoom call with a guy named "Dr. Jeff" who looks like he just stepped out of an audition for *The Bachelor*. Your first move is always the same: Show them what they're dealing with. But do not—I repeat, *do not*—tell them your life story. You are not writing a memoir. Doctors, even the good ones, have the attention span of a squirrel, and if you start explaining how your fatigue started in 2013 after you had your second kid and your gluten sensitivity kicked in during your kombucha cleanse, you've already lost them. What you need to take with you is a bulleted list of your top symptoms, up to fifteen in total. For example:

- Fatigue
- Brain fog
- Constipation
- Hair thinning
- Cold intolerance
- Weight gain
- Depression
- Dry skin
- Brittle nails
- Low libido
- Anxiety
- Mood swings
- Joint pain
- Irregular periods
- Poor sleep

Don't explain your symptoms, describe them, or apologize for them. Hand the list over and say, "This is what I'm experiencing, and I want to get to the bottom of it."

2. Know What You Want
You're not begging for someone to figure you out; you're acting as the CEO of your own body, with lab results and a clear direction. Think

about your intention before you go in. What is it that you intend to make happen here?

If you're not on thyroid meds yet but you've taken this book to heart and done your due diligence—you've looked at your labs, you've seen that your free T3 is low, your reverse T3 is high, and your TSH is nudging toward dysfunction—guess what? You're not there to discuss "if" you need treatment. You're there to discuss "how" to get the treatment you need. Thyroid hormone replacement isn't a maybe, it's a must. And because you know what these markers mean, you're already ahead of 99 percent of patients (and frankly, 80 percent of doctors).

If you're starting at the very beginning and know you need lab work—the *right* labs—because you strongly suspect thyroid dysfunction, you need to start there and ask for a complete lab panel with *all* the labs I outlined and discussed in chapter 5. And remember the golden rule: If your doctor says no to ordering all the labs you are requesting, it's time to get a new doctor.

3. Read the Room and Lead the Conversation

Let's say you already have your lab results in hand, and here's what you know.

- Your reverse T3 is elevated.
- Your free T3 is low.
- Your TSH is high.
- Your free T4 is approaching the too-high zone.

Now let's say your doctor pulls out a prescription pad and scribbles, "100 mcg of T4."

This is when you speak up: "Actually, I've done some research on this, and based on my current labs, especially with my reverse T3 being at 18 ng/dL, I'd feel more comfortable starting on a lower dose of T4.

Maybe 25 to 50 micrograms, max. I'm also open to adding T3, since my free T3 is low, and I know that's the active hormone that every cell in my body needs."

Boom. Simple. Direct. No drama. No fear.

You are not asking permission. You are communicating what you need to feel safe and supported in your treatment.

And if your provider throws out one of the greatest hits such as:

"T3 causes heart attacks."

"You don't need T3. T4 converts just fine."

"We don't test reverse T3. That's not necessary."

Then you smile, thank them for their time, and leave. That's not the doctor for you.

4. Push for Optimization, Not Just Treatment

If you're already on thyroid meds but they're not working, or if you've been stuck on the same low 25 mcg dose of T3 for years with no relief, you have the same right to rework your plan as someone who is starting from scratch. This is not just a "live with it" situation, and you now have more information and firepower.

Tell your doctor, "I appreciate what we've tried so far, but I'm still not feeling better. Based on my labs and my symptoms, I'd like to explore different medication options or combinations so I can feel well." Short. Direct. You're not insulting your provider's plan, you're asking them to expand it.

Or "My labs show that my free T3 is still low, nowhere near the optimal range. I know that every cell in my body has a receptor site for T3, not T4, and I'm still symptomatic. So I'd like to increase my T3 dose slightly, maybe 5 micrograms more twice a day, and see how I respond."

If you have a provider who is very T4 only, try countering their resistance with facts: "The American Academy of Anti-Aging Medicine reports that T4-only treatment is effective for just 2 percent of people with hypothyroidism. That means the other 98 percent need either a T4/T3 combination or even just T3 only, if they're not converting well. Since T4 hasn't worked for me, I'd like to try one of these other options."

You can also lay out your own lab numbers: "Right now, I'm on 100 micrograms of T4. My reverse T3 is 18 ng/dL, which is high. My free T3 is at the bottom of the range. That tells me I'm not converting well. I'd like to lower my T4 and add some T3."

Then add this: "I want this to be a partnership. I'm not here to go rogue. I just want to work with someone who understands that one-size-fits-all treatment doesn't work, and I'm not okay staying sick when there are other options. I'm happy to track my progress and keep the lines of communication open so we can fine-tune as we go."

In this way, you've shifted from being a passive patient to taking the lead. You're not being combative, you're hiring someone to do a job. You're paying them, whether it's with insurance, co-pays, or your own wallet. You're the client, not a charity case.

You're not asking for something outrageous; you're asking for a measurable, trackable adjustment based on clear evidence and clear symptoms. If the provider is worth their salt, they'll listen. If they're stuck in the old-school mindset of "low and slow and don't touch the T3," you'll know then and there that it's time to level up to someone better.

5. Don't Settle for Baby Doses

If your doctor finally agrees to T3 but prescribes you only 5 mcg once a day and says, "Let's see how that goes," is that a win?

Yes and no. Five mcg is a baby dose. That's like handing you a single ice cube when you're stranded in the desert. Five mcg once a day is a good place to start, and some very sensitive people need to start even lower, at 2.5 mcg once a day. But the reality is that most people don't see their symptoms start to turn around until they are on, at minimum, 15 to 20 mcg *twice* a day, and some people aren't optimized until they reach 50 or even 100 mcg twice a day. There is a huge variation in what works for people, so you need a titration strategy. You need to know where you're headed. You're aiming for optimization, not just "Well, at least we tried."

Here's what you can say: "I appreciate that you're open to T3, but I want to work toward a dose that truly changes how I feel. I'm fine starting low, but my goal is to optimize based on both my labs and my symptoms. Can we make a plan for when we'll retest and reevaluate to see if I need a higher dose?"

The rate at which patients can progress their dosing will vary, and I guide everyone differently based on their symptoms and response to the T3. Some people can go up another 5 mcg after as little as five to seven days, as long as they aren't feeling anxious or jittery or experiencing any other side effects. Other patients need to go more slowly, and we progress them every two to four weeks. If you do experience side effects, it does *not* mean that you cannot tolerate T3 at higher levels or that you need to stop progressing—it just means that you need to go at a slower pace. So you can back down from the 5 mcg increase, hold at that level for a week or so, and then try increasing by 2.5 mcg instead. There is no rush. Yes, you want to feel better as soon as possible, but it's better to give your body time to adjust to the medication so that you can ultimately reach those higher levels where you will be optimized and feel fantastic.

In my experience, four weeks is plenty of time to know what a specific dose is going to do. If after four weeks, you're still symptomatic and your labs show that your free T3 is still below the upper quadrant of the "normal" range, tell your provider that you'd like to try increasing the dose by another 5 mcg.

• • •

Above all, when you're talking to your doctor, be clear. Be confident. This is not the moment to let outdated rules or myths keep you sick. You're not there to be "managed." You're there to get your life back.

How to Get T3: The Quick Script

Getting a provider to prescribe T3 is one of the biggest and most common challenges faced by thyroid patients, so I want to call it out here and give you exactly what you need to make your case. As long as you know your lab results, you can follow the formula below and succeed. You don't have to walk in knowing the exact dose you need; just hit your provider with these facts:

- T4 only isn't working for you.

- Your labs show poor conversion.

- You need T3 in the mix.

- Reducing T4 can help lower reverse T3.

- You want to develop a collaborative plan.

- You deserve treatment that's designed for you, not the "average" patient.

   If your doctor won't have the T3 conversation, keep looking. Whether it takes one try or six, there are providers out there who either know how to do this or are willing to learn. Have the conversation. Use your voice. This is your health. Your life. And you are done waiting.

Chapter 8

Can I Heal My Thyroid Naturally?

Here's another question I hear every day: "Can I heal my thyroid naturally?"

I know what's behind this, but I can't say I understand it. Almost everyone will take a vitamin supplement without hesitation. They know it makes them feel better. They pick up the bottle, take it daily, and move on. But if something comes in an amber pill bottle from the pharmacy, suddenly they get the heebie-jeebies. It's as though some invisible line exists and taking a prescription means we're old or caving in to something that goes against our core beliefs.

I know you *want* to believe that if you just sprinkle the right adaptogen powder into your smoothie, follow a certain influencer's protocol, detox your liver with an overpriced binder, and meditate under the full moon, you can reverse your thyroid symptoms and feel like yourself again without ever having to pick up a medication bottle. But I'm here to tell you the truth because I want you to get better: What you need is hormone replacement.

Why is replacing the hormones our bodies can no longer make considered "unnatural," while vitamin D gets a free pass? Vitamin D is also a hormone, vitamin D supplements are produced by labs and manufacturers, and we don't debate taking them or declare, "I'm going natural, so I'll just stand outside in January to get some sun and hope for the best." We take it without shame or resistance.

Thyroid hormone should be no different. Every form of thyroid medication is bioidentical, meaning that it matches exactly what your body can no longer produce. The only difference is that the hormones you get with a prescription are synthesized in a lab; the molecular components are the same as if they had been produced by you. Yet I still hear women say they want to "do it naturally," as if there's a badge of honor for avoiding a prescription. Meanwhile, they're dealing with brain fog, joint pain, hot flashes, zero libido, thinning hair, skin problems, and an expanding waistline.

I'm not dismissing your desire to keep things natural. I'm asking you to think about what "natural" really means. Insulin is a hormone, too. No one tells a person with type 1 diabetes to "fix it naturally" with cinnamon and sunshine. Without insulin, they wouldn't survive. It's not an option, it's basic biology.

I know what you're thinking: "I'm not going to die without thyroid hormone." Okay. Maybe not today. But over time? You will suffer. Your brain function and metabolism will deteriorate. Your cardiovascular system will start breaking down. Your immune system will weaken. You'll gain weight that won't budge, stop getting restful sleep, become uninterested in sex, lose your hair, see your skin age more quickly, and lose your drive, joy, and memory.

But hey . . . at least you're living "naturally," right?

I want to be crystal clear with you on this. If you are in the early stages of thyroid dysfunction, your blood work numbers are close to optimal, and you've just started noticing symptoms, then fine, give the natural route a try. Clean up your diet. Take the right supplements. Support your adrenals. Sleep better. Hydrate. Get outside in the sunshine. I'm all for it. In the early days, reversal with lifestyle changes can be possible, and I'll talk more about how you do this in the pages ahead.

But if you've been struggling for months or years with the full lineup of symptoms, you've already burned through precious time and exhausted your body trying to feel better without treating a thyroid that is no longer doing its job. If your body isn't making enough thyroid hormone, replacing it isn't giving up; it's giving yourself a fighting chance.

Sometimes patients come to me who have made peace with the idea of hormone replacement but are stuck in the "only natural desiccated thyroid" mindset. They tell me that they want only Armour Thyroid, for example, or NP Thyroid, because those brands have "natural" on the label and that makes them feel safer somehow. If this sounds like you, remember what I said at the start of chapter 6: My favorite thyroid medication is the one that works for *you*. Unlike many functional practitioners, I'm not married to natural desiccated thyroid (NDT) products, and you shouldn't be, either. I've seen them work miracles. I've also seen them increase reverse T3, trigger autoimmune flares, and make women feel worse. Sometimes compounded T3 is the turning point for someone. Sometimes a biosynthetic combo is the sweet spot. You need to be open-minded, because it all depends on your unique biochemistry.

Here's my advice: Stop thinking of "synthetic" as a dirty word. It's not. Synthroid, Cytomel, levothyroxine—these medications are produced by replicating a biosynthetic process that happens inside your body, and they are biologically identical to what your body should be making. Yes, they're made in a lab, but they function just like the hormones your thyroid used to produce. I don't want you to insist on staying in a "natural" box and then wonder why you still feel like garbage.

At the end of the day, what really matter are results and quality of life. What matters is getting your energy, brain function, sex drive, metabolism, and joy back—all things that should be yours by right. That's the kind of "natural" I care about.

So . . . Can I Fix My Thyroid Naturally?

Yes, it's possible, if you are lucky and catch the problem early. And—and I really want you to hear me say this—*if* you are not already drowning in a deluge of symptoms.

Let's say you are one of the fortunate ones reading this book in the early stages of thyroid problems. You might have one or two symptoms, nothing debilitating or soul sucking. You are still functioning, still living your life. You've had a full thyroid panel run—and yes, I mean the entire panel, not just TSH—and your labs look pretty good, close to optimal. Maybe you have a few antibodies creeping in. Maybe your free T3 is just a touch low, a few points under where you want it to be. You are in the gray zone: nothing clinically disastrous but no longer optimal.

If you fit the profile above, here is an eight-point plan of what you can do naturally to support your thyroid. I will go deeper into all these approaches in part III, but here are the highlights.

1. **Take vitamins.** Your thyroid runs on nutrients, not hopes and prayers. You need vitamin D3 (a hormone, remember), B vitamins, selenium, magnesium, and most of all, iodine. Your thyroid needs iodine to make both T4 and T3, and every cell in your body, not just your thyroid, uses iodine. It is the single most important supplement you can take.

2. **Take black cumin seed oil.** This remarkable supplement has evidence-backed support for improvement of Hashimoto's thyroiditis. Studies show that it can lower thyroid antibodies, reduce inflammation, ease fatigue and joint pain, and help with many other autoimmune-related symptoms.[1]

3. **Take T2.** T2 is a lesser-known but incredibly powerful thyroid hormone that supports T4 to T3 conversion, boosts metabolism, and increases cellular energy without spiking cortisol or altering TSH.[2] T2 also decreases inflammation throughout the body, turns on genes that prevent fat accumulation, and reduces oxidative stress, which helps protect your cells from damage.[3] Best of all, it's available over the counter. I'll talk more about T2 in chapter 10.

4. **Eat clean.** If you are going to try to heal your thyroid naturally by eating clean, you have to go all in. This is not about eating clean Monday through Friday and then loading up on margaritas and nachos over the weekend. Garbage in equals garbage out. Processed food, sugar, and seed oils are all highly inflammatory. They sabotage your thyroid, spike your insulin, and crank up reverse T3. Even a

small amount can set off a cascade of inflammation that grinds your thyroid to a halt. If you are serious about going natural, that means eating whole foods. Period.

5. **Move.** You have to move, and I'm not just talking about yoga or a casual walk around the block. Movement is about getting your heart rate up, your blood moving, and your metabolism firing. Studies show that strength training or resistance training with weights is the best way to build muscle, burn fat, regulate your insulin, and promote detoxification.[4] Cardio, on the other hand, can tax your body in ways that are counterproductive. Being physically active in the *right* way is not optional when you are rebooting your hormones.

6. **Get enough high-quality sleep.** You are not a "night owl." If you are not in bed by 10:00 p.m., you are missing the deep restorative time for repair and healing that your body needs. One of the fastest ways to sabotage T4 to T3 conversion is to jack up your insulin and cortisol,[5] and sugar and sleep deprivation will do just that. If you can eliminate these two things, you will be healthier than 90 percent of the population.

7. **Manage your stress.** If your cortisol is either tanked or running high around the clock, nothing else you do for your thyroid is going to work. No supplement, no amount of clean eating, and no fancy biohack will help you outrun a cortisol crisis. You cannot sporadically meditate your way out of it. You must actively manage your stress every single day.

8. **Improve your gut health.** Your gut is ground zero for metabolism, inflammation, nutrient absorption, and immune function, as well as a critical site for T4 to T3 conversion. If your gut is a mess, your thyroid will be, too. Everything I have talked about, including food, sleep, and stress, loops back to gut health. Eating fermented foods such as sauerkraut and kimchi, taking digestive enzymes with your meals, eliminating processed foods and sugars, and taking collagen and colostrum supplements will all help keep your gut working properly. Sometimes there are deeper issues that need to

be addressed with a gut specialist, such as small intestine bacterial overgrowth (SIBO) or *H. pylori* infection, that are beyond the scope of this book. Just know that your gut needs some love if you're going to go the natural route.

Now Here's the Reality Check

If you've caught your condition early, if you're not too deep in dysfunction, if your labs are decent and your symptoms are mild, you can do all these things and *maybe* avoid having to take medication. But I will not sugarcoat it for you: If you're half-assing it—still sporadically eating processed food, staying up past midnight every night, and just "trying a few things" while watching your life unravel—you're not healing anything. You're stalling. And you're suffering unnecessarily.

And if things get worse? If you've done all these things and your numbers still plummet, your symptoms explode, and your life starts to fall apart, it's time to stop fighting the idea of hormone replacement and start taking steps to get your life back.

This book is about real healing—sustainable, evidence-based, freedom-to-live-your-life kind of healing. Sometimes that starts with a supplement. Sometimes it starts with a script. Sometimes it starts with finally saying out loud, "I'm not okay, and I'm ready to stop pretending that I am."

You don't owe it to anyone to "stay natural." You owe it to yourself to feel better.

PART III

Breaking Bad(ass): Game-Changing New Habits to Support Your Thyroid Health

Chapter 9

Supplement like You Mean It

I've never been the type of practitioner who believes in loading people down with supplements or saying that they are a magical cure for all their ailments. Nor am I someone who pooh-poohs prescription medication, as I have made clear. Thyroid hormone replacement and bioidentical hormones play a significant and crucial role in thyroid care. They can benefit your body in powerful ways and be nothing short of game changing when used properly. Supplements are meant to support, not replace medications. But if used strategically, supplements can correct deficiencies or enhance pathways that need a little help, improving your thyroid function and promoting hormonal harmony throughout your body.

It is the Wild West of supplements out there, and it can be overwhelming, especially when influencers are shouting that you must have this and can't live without that. A patient once came to me for an initial visit with a list of supplements she was taking that was two pages long. And, like 80 percent of the people I meet, she couldn't explain or give a specific reason for why she was taking half of them. The most common explanation I hear from my patients is that another doctor told them to take a certain supplement or that they read about it on a thyroid blog somewhere. But my first rule of supplements is that you always need to know what problem or imbalance a particular product is trying to address. Otherwise, how will you know if it is working?

The other problem that I see patients encounter when trying to navigate the supplement universe is that the industry on the whole has little regulation and not all products are created equal. There's a moment in Chris Bell's 2008 documentary about anabolic steroids, *Bigger, Stronger, Faster*, that shows exactly how easy it is to counterfeit supplements. In one clip, Bell picks up day laborers from the side of the road, takes them to his apartment, spreads out empty capsules on the kitchen table, mixes some unknown powders in a big bowl as though he is baking a cake, and has the workers, with no regulations and no oversight, fill the capsules, bottle them, and slap on a professional-looking label. Just like that, he has a supplement ready to sell on Amazon. That might sound extreme, but it is real. It shows you how unregulated this space can be.

When I ask patients where they purchase their supplements, they typically say Walmart, Costco, or Amazon. I don't want to knock these companies, because I sell my line of products on Amazon, too. But my strong feeling, which I've been saying for decades, is that you should buy directly from companies that are owned by individuals rather than large corporations whenever possible. When you buy supplements from huge corporate entities that mass-produce for big-box stores, your chances of getting lower-quality ingredients go way up, especially when brands have sold out to companies such as Nestlé or pharmaceutical giants such as Bayer. The quality is just not the same as when someone owns and runs their company themselves. Back in my bodybuilding days, long before I dreamed of having my own supplement line, I bought my sports supplements from people such as Lee Labrada and Rich Gaspari, individuals whose names and reputations were on the line every time someone opened a bottle. That's the difference. And that's why *where* you buy your supplements matters just as much as what you take.

If you're someone whose supplement list has ballooned over the course of your thyroid journey, I'm here to help you streamline it. You don't need a two-page list of expensive products, no matter what the influencers say. What follows is what I lovingly call my "No Duh" supplement list, the key vitamins, minerals, and other nutrients you need to support your thyroid and all the other systems around it every single day. I'm totally dating myself with that phrase, pulling it from my childhood in the 1980s, when we would say "No duh" to anything that was blatantly obvious. As in "The sky is blue." "No duh." With these key supplements, there are no questions, no debate, no sketchy TikTok trends. They are scientifically proven and absolutely useful, and if you want to bolster your thyroid health, taking them is nonnegotiable.

Iodine

In the functional medicine world, opinions are split on iodine, but the split is not fifty-fifty. It's more like seventy-thirty, where 70 percent of functional practitioners, including me, are pro-iodine and recognize its benefits. The other 30 percent are anti-iodine, and those folks are scaring the bejesus out of people about taking it. Here's the problem: Many anti-iodine practitioners haven't done enough research to form a science-backed, well-educated opinion, but they are still out there spreading fear that iodine is dangerous, it can do more harm than good, and you should avoid it. But we don't make good decisions when we come from a place of fear. We make great decisions based on science.

There are entire books that break down iodine's history and benefits and make arguments for and against its use. The reality is that iodine has been used since World War II for treating everything from gunshot wounds to the common cold. It is antiviral and antibacterial and kills off pathogens. It helps with fibrocystic breasts and endometrial fibroids.[1] And in the thyroid, as we have seen, iodine plays a crucial role. It aids in the production of all four thyroid hormones and even supports the conversion of inactive T4 to active T3.[2]

Some of iodine's bad reputation comes from confusion between iodine supplementation and radioactive iodine treatment. Iodine, the nutrient we get through dietary sources such as seafood, dairy products, eggs, and iodized salt, is essential. Your thyroid can't do its jobs without it. On the other hand, radioactive iodine is a medical therapy used to destroy thyroid tissue in cases of Graves' disease, hyperthyroidism, or thyroid cancer. Because the thyroid naturally soaks up iodine, when a radioactive isotope is administered, the gland absorbs it and the radiation kills thyroid cells. That's the point of the treatment. It's helpful in the right context but not the same thing as nutritional iodine. One supports thyroid health, the other wipes it out. Big difference.

The confusion, however, doesn't end there. Millions of people take iodine supplements safely every day, but some practitioners have irresponsibly prescribed very high doses. Too much iodine can overstimulate the thyroid and push a person into hyperthyroidism,[3] or, in rare cases, trigger a thyroid storm, which is essentially hyperthyroidism on steroids and dangerous for the heart. But those cases are rare. Most knowledgeable practitioners are not going to put someone on massive doses of iodine without careful titration. Still, it takes only one or two bad outcomes to create fear. A handful of cases, and suddenly there are books and blogs warning people not to touch iodine or even eat iodine-containing foods. Based on the research, that kind of blanket fear is, frankly, ludicrous.

As we saw in chapter 3, iodine is part of the halogen family, which also includes bromine, chlorine, and fluorine. Unlike iodine, the other three halogens are toxins that can wreak havoc on the thyroid due to their similar molecular structure. But it is not just your thyroid that is at risk; every cell in your body has receptor sites for iodine. If you don't have enough iodine in your body to fill those sites, the three toxic halogens will step in and take its place.[4] If you don't nourish your cells with iodine, you can expect them to be filled with chlorine, bromine, and fluorine instead.

And as we have seen, these toxins are everywhere. Chlorine is in your water system. Bromine is in your clothing, furniture, carpets, and plastics. Fluorine, in the form of fluoride, is in your drinking water and your toothpaste, and if you are a child of the 1980s or '90s, you probably remember those little pink fluoride pills the dentist used to hand out.

We know from research that high levels of fluoride exposure, particularly from drinking water, can negatively impact thyroid function and increase the risk of hypothyroidism.[5] This is because fluoride is so similar to iodine in terms of its molecular structure that it interferes with iodine uptake by thyroid cells, which leads to decreased production and lower

levels of T3 and T4. Research also links higher levels of fluoride in drinking water to higher TSH levels,[6] which, as we know, are an indication
that your body is working overtime to get your thyroid to respond. If you
are already low in iodine due to nutritional insufficiencies, it gets worse.
Studies on children have shown that when fluoride exposure occurs in
the context of a natural iodine deficiency, there is a higher frequency of
both functional problems and structural changes in the thyroid gland as
well as intellectual challenges.[7]

Fortunately, regular supplementation with iodine can prevent these
problems and support your thyroid. Sometimes patients with hypothyroidism even feel the benefits of iodine supplementation physically. This
is because low iodine also contributes to elevated reverse T3, your anti-
thyroid hormone, the one that puts you into survival mode or human
dormancy. But when we add iodine to your system, reverse T3 levels
drop[8] and patients who might not even be fully optimized on T3 feel a
shift.

There are two types of iodine used in supplementation, potassium
iodide and nascent iodine. Potassium iodide has been used for decades
in iodized salt and certain medical treatments. Nascent iodine is a newer
form that the body can absorb and utilize more efficiently. I spent years
studying both to determine which was best to support the body and the
thyroid, and I decided on nascent iodine because the literature shows
it is highly bioavailable, meaning easy for the body to absorb and use.[9]
It's also a gentler form of iodine, so the risks of side effects or of pushing
someone into a hyperthyroid state are much lower.[10] That matters, especially for those who are already coping with symptoms and trying to
correct years of being undertreated.

Normally, iodine is found in a bonded form in which two iodine
molecules are stuck together, called I_2. But this molecular structure is
difficult for the body to break apart and use. In the past, doctors used
potassium iodide combined with I_2 to treat iodine deficiency. That is
also the basis of iodized salt, which contains small amounts of potassium
iodide. The problem is that potassium iodide can sometimes trigger in-

flammation in the thyroid (thyroiditis).[11] On top of that, many people today are avoiding table salt or switching to natural salts that do not contain added iodine, leaving them vulnerable to deficiency.

Nascent iodine, also known as atomic iodine, solves all these problems. It is made by taking molecular iodine and exposing it to a strong magnetic field, which splits it into individual atoms. These single iodine atoms are in a highly energized state, ready to be absorbed and used by your cells. That is what makes nascent iodine so effective. There's no conversion required and no waste, just direct support for your thyroid. It also helps with metabolism, mood, energy, immune health, cognitive function, and overall hormonal balance.

No matter what form of iodine you use, you always want to look at what it is mixed with. Nascent iodine supplements come in liquid form. If the base is glycerin, that is a cheaper version and can blunt nascent iodine's effects in the body. You want to make sure that the base is alcohol, which allows for better absorption and utilization.

When taking iodine, start low and slow, no matter which version you are using. I tell all my patients to start with a single drop of liquid iodine in a small shot glass of water. Add a little apple cider vinegar to cut the taste and a pinch of salt to help your body utilize the iodine and prevent jittery side effects. You can increase by one drop per day until you reach your tolerance level. If you are wondering how to gauge your tolerance, trust me, you will know it. You will get an icky, sticky feeling, a kind of jittery, wired sensation as though you just slammed three energy drinks back to back. That is your body saying, "Okay, hold up." That is your signal to return to the dose you were at the day before, the one that made you feel good, clear, and energized without crossing the line into overstimulation. This response from your body doesn't mean you'll *never* be able to increase your dose; it just means that you are adjusting and right now, you are at a solid level of iodine intake. As your body acclimates to it, you may be able to increase slowly again in the future.

I take iodine every day. My dose is around sixty drops of my Iodine

Fixxr supplement in water. I just slam it down and move on with my day. But if I am traveling or feel as though I'm getting sick, I take the same dose twice a day. I find it helps protect me against colds and viruses and gives my immune system an extra edge. Here are recommendations depending on which protocol you choose.

Iodine Protocol
Your goal is to find your optimal dose between 6 and 50 mg per day. Follow the product's instructions for dosing, and go slowly. Slow titration keeps you in tune with what your body needs and prevents overstimulation.

Iodine Fixxr Protocol
Begin with one drop per day in one ounce or less of water. Increase by one drop daily while paying attention to how you feel. Most people either feel nothing or notice a gentle lift in energy. Again, your goal is to find the dose that works for you, somewhere between 6 and 50 mg per day.

Magnesium

Magnesium is involved in so many bodily functions that it is hard to overstate its importance. It is essential to over three hundred biochemical reactions, including the production of adenosine triphosphate (ATP). It also boosts metabolism, supports muscle relaxation, helps with sleep and stress, calms the nervous system, regulates blood pressure, enhances nerve function, and, as you may have guessed, is critical for thyroid health.

Magnesium facilitates iodine uptake by your thyroid and acts as a cofactor for the enzymes type 1 and type 2 deiodinase (D1 and D2), which convert T4 to T3. It's not surprising, then, that low magnesium levels are linked to an increased risk of thyroid issues, including Hashimoto's.[12] Stress can also be a factor. Science has shown that there's a strong link among magnesium levels, adrenal function, and thyroid function.[13]

Most thyroid patients tend to be more sensitive to stress, which means they burn through magnesium more quickly than the average person does.[14] To complicate things further, thyroid dysfunction directly impacts how your body handles magnesium. An underactive or overactive thyroid can alter how your kidneys regulate magnesium,[15] affecting how much is excreted from your body and how much is retained. Even if you are getting enough magnesium from supplements, your body might not be able to hold on to it if your thyroid is off.

That's why it is so important for thyroid patients to be intentional about magnesium support. It is not just about getting enough, it is about making sure your body can use it well. Unfortunately, thanks to modern farming practices and soil depletion, the magnesium content in our food is lower than it used to be, which means that few of us get enough naturally, even if we are eating clean, whole foods. For all these reasons, thyroid patients often require higher amounts of magnesium than can be obtained through diet alone to maintain balance and feel their best.

There are many different forms of magnesium, and they are not all created equal. The form you take will make a difference in how well your body absorbs it and what benefits you derive. The most common form on the market is **magnesium citrate**, which is often used to relieve constipation due to its natural laxative effect. Research has shown that magnesium citrate may also help increase bone mineral density, especially in postmenopausal women,[16] an added bonus. It also has decent bioavailability, meaning that your body absorbs it more efficiently than other forms such as magnesium oxide.

Magnesium oxide is often overlooked because it has a lower bioavailability when blood levels are measured, but it still provides meaningful benefits. It is particularly helpful for supporting digestion, easing heartburn, reducing indigestion, and relieving occasional constipation.[17] Magnesium oxide draws water into the intestines, which can gently promote regularity and reduce that heavy, sluggish feeling that many thyroid patients experience when their digestion slows down. It also supports overall gut motility and can help keep things moving when stress, low thyroid function, or certain medications back everything up. While it may not be the form you should rely on for deep cellular replenishment, it can play an important supportive role in digestive comfort and regularity.

Magnesium glycinate is a good option for thyroid support as well as calming the nervous system. The magnesium is highly bioavailable and bound to the amino acid glycine, which makes it especially helpful for anxiety, depression, sleep support, and even digestion.[18] This form promotes relaxation, so it is great for winding down in the evening or easing stress throughout the day. It is gentle on the stomach, nonlaxative, and works well for daily use.

I feel, however, that **magnesium malate** is the standout form for thyroid patients, and it is the one I recommend most often to patients who are dealing with low energy, chronic fatigue, muscle pain, or fibromyalgia-like symptoms. The malate portion comes from malic acid, which is directly involved in the Krebs cycle, your body's energy production engine. Thus, you are both getting magnesium support for your thyroid and fueling your mitochondria. Magnesium malate can also improve exercise performance, boost mood, enhance sleep, reduce muscle tightness, and support deep cellular energy production.[19]

Different forms of magnesium serve different purposes, so it is important to choose the one that best matches your body's needs. You can also look for a magnesium blend that contains more than one type, such as Quad Magnesium by the Fixxr.

Magnesium Protocol (Choose One Type)
Magnesium citrate: 200–400 mg per day
Magnesium oxide: 250–500 mg per day
Magnesium glycinate: 200–600 mg per day
Magnesium malate: 200–600 mg per day

Quad Magnesium by the Fixxr Protocol

Take two capsules at night to support deep sleep, calm your nervous system, relax muscles, and improve stress resilience. You can also take them during the day if that works better for you.

B Vitamins

B vitamins are some of the hardest-working nutrients in your body, and they are deeply tied to thyroid function. They help your cells turn the food you eat into usable energy, support red blood cell production, maintain a healthy nervous system, and keep your methylation pathways running.[20] Methylation is the cellular process that turns genes on and off, and it affects detoxification and hormone balance. Additionally, several B vitamins, including B_2, B_6, B_9, and B_{12}, are directly involved in thyroid hormone production and activation.

Even if your thyroid medication is optimized on paper, you may still feel chronically tired, foggy, weak, and depressed if you are low in B vitamins. Low B_{12} in particular is incredibly common in patients with Hashimoto's, because autoimmune-related gastritis and low stomach acid can make it more difficult for the body to absorb B_{12} through the digestive tract.[21] Low B_{12} can also mimic or magnify hypothyroid symptoms, including numbness and tingling in the hands and feet, memory problems, low mood, and profound fatigue.[22] So making sure that you are getting enough B vitamins to compensate for any malabsorption is key to eliminating symptoms and feeling your best.

This is why I include a high-quality B complex, such as my B Fixxr, on my "No Duh" supplement list as part of basic thyroid support. When your cells are replete with B vitamins, they respond better to thyroid hormone, your energy production improves, your thyroid hormone production improves,[23] and your whole system runs more smoothly. You can take individual B vitamins or look for a good B complex that includes B_{12} and other Bs (B_1, B_3, B_5, and B_7) and approximates the targets in the following suggested protocol.

B Vitamin Protocol

Vitamin B_2 (riboflavin/riboflavin-5-phosphate): 25–100 mg per day

Vitamin B_6 (pyridoxine or P5P): 25–100 mg per day

Vitamin B_9 (methylfolate of folinic acid): 400–800 mcg per day

Vitamin B_{12} (methylcobalamin or adenosylcobalamin/ hydroxocobalamin): 1,000–5,000 mcg per day

B Fixxr Protocol

Take one serving per day to support thyroid hormone production, energy, red blood cell formation, methylation, and neurotransmitter balance.

Vitamin D_3

Yes, it is popularly called a vitamin, but as I already pointed out, vitamin D is really a hormone. We obtain vitamin D through exposure to sunlight and through food, but once it is in our bodies, it is converted to its active hormonal form, calcitriol, by the liver and kidneys. It then circulates throughout the body, acting on cells and various biochemical processes just as other hormones do.

Your thyroid gland has receptors for active vitamin D, which means that this unsung hormone has a direct impact on thyroid function and health. Vitamin D helps regulate thyroid hormone production by increasing levels of type 2 deiodinase,[24] one of the enzymes responsible for converting T4 to T3. Numerous studies have also shown that vitamin D calms the immune system and reduces the anti-thyroid antibodies TPO and TgAb.[25] It suppresses inflammation and supports the development of T regulatory cells, the cells that prevent your immune system from attacking your own body.[26] That is a big deal if you are dealing with an autoimmune condition such as Hashimoto's or Graves' disease. On the flip side, low vitamin D levels are linked to a higher risk of thyroid-related autoimmune diseases, meaning that supplementing has clear preventive benefits as well.

Beyond autoimmune disorders, research shows a link between low levels of vitamin D and more aggressive forms of thyroid cancer.[27] This connection is not all that surprising when you realize how crucial vitamin D is for immune system regulation and inflammation control in general. When your vitamin D level is low, your body has a harder time managing inflammation and detecting abnormal cell growth, both of which play major roles in cancer development and progression. In the case of thyroid cancer, insufficient vitamin D may not only increase your risk but also influence how quickly the disease advances and how your body responds to it.

In addition to helping prevent autoimmune disease and cancer, vitamin D plays a powerful role in supporting your adrenal glands and balancing your sex hormones,[28] two systems that are almost always disrupted when the thyroid goes off track. When thyroid function declines, it often triggers a cascade of hormonal imbalances, and vitamin D helps support and stabilize the entire network.

As you can see, vitamin D supports far more in our bodies than just bone health. It is a foundational hormone that quietly works behind the scenes to keep your body in balance. Yet most people are walking around deficient in vitamin D without realizing it. Most of us do not come close to the 600 IU daily recommended for women over the age of twenty, and I would argue that that amount is far too low.

That is why vitamin D, in the form of vitamin D_3, is what I call a daily nonnegotiable. Especially if you are dealing with thyroid issues, adrenal fatigue, low mood, hormonal swings, or immune challenges, this is one supplement that belongs in your routine every single day. It is doing more than you realize to keep your body and thyroid resilient, well regulated, and ready to heal.

Vitamin D_3 Protocol

Take 10,000 IU per day together with 2 mg of vitamin K_2 for proper absorption and safety. Vitamin D_3 is fat-soluble, so it should be taken with a meal that contains healthy fats.

Vit D Fixxr Protocol

Includes 10,000 IU per day together with 2 mg of vitamin K. Take one capsule daily and include a source of dietary fat to help with uptake.

Black Cumin Seed Oil

Black cumin seed oil is one of the most powerful and underrated supplements, although this might be the first time you are hearing about it. It is derived from *Nigella sativa*, a plant that has been used in traditional medicine for centuries. And its benefits are mind-blowing.

Black cumin seed oil helps lower antibodies across the board in all autoimmune conditions, treats arthritis and other inflammatory disorders, supports weight loss, improves glucose regulation, and even helps protect against cancer.[29] Its active ingredient is thymoquinone, a phytochemical loaded with antioxidant properties. Note that black cumin is entirely different from the cumin that you cook with. We'll dive into all black cumin seed oil's amazing uses, but first, let me tell you what it does for the thyroid.

When it comes to treating Hashimoto's thyroiditis, black cumin seed oil has a growing body of data behind it. It has been shown to lower autoimmune antibodies, reduce systemic inflammation, and modulate the immune response.[30] In particular, it targets thyroid peroxidase antibodies,[31] a key marker of Hashimoto's. Anecdotally, in my practice, we have seen patients on black cumin seed oil who have completely reversed their Hashimoto's, putting it into remission and lowering their antibodies to nearly zero. Other patient reports have shown drops of over 200 units in antibody levels. That is not a subtle effect. It is significant.

Thymoquinone, the active compound, provides impressive protection and support for thyroid health. Its strong antioxidant properties help combat oxidative stress,[32] an imbalance of free radicals throughout the body that can damage cells, proteins, and DNA and contribute to thyroid cell damage. By reducing your body's oxidative load, thymoquinone helps preserve thyroid tissue and function. It also plays a direct role in improving hormone balance, and studies show that it can lower elevated TSH while boosting both T4 and T3,[33] helping your body restore proper thyroid function and control.

Beyond thyroid support, black cumin seed oil has clear benefits for weight management, which makes all of us happy. Research shows that it can help reduce weight, body mass index, and waist circumference.[34] It is also well known among patients with type 2 diabetes for its ability to help regulate blood sugar. Multiple studies have found that individuals taking black cumin seed oil had significantly lower fasting glucose levels and improved insulin sensitivity compared to those taking a placebo.[35] It appears to help reset your metabolism, which, as we know, directly impacts your thyroid function.

What makes black cumin seed oil so valuable and exciting is that it addresses several systems at once. It supports the entire HPT axis, eases inflammation, aids in weight loss, and helps manage blood sugar, all of which are interconnected in anyone dealing with thyroid issues. And its benefits do not stop there. It has also been shown to reduce rheumatoid arthritis inflammation markers as well as arthritis symptoms such as swollen joints.[36] It helps with sinusitis and allergies[37] due to its antimicrobial, anti-inflammatory, and antihistaminic properties, blocking your body's histamines naturally to help relieve allergy symptoms. It is also an analgesic, meaning that it reduces pain without causing drowsiness.[38] It supports heart health by lowering lipid counts[39] in people with hyperlipidemia, and some studies have shown that it may help lower high blood pressure as well.[40]

And then there is the big one, the one I would not even mention if it did not have legitimate scientific backing: Black cumin seed oil has anti-cancer activity. It is almost impossible for any supplement to claim direct anti-cancer benefits, because the moment a company tries to make that claim without proof, it gets shut down. But in the case of black cumin seed oil, we can talk about it because there are peer-reviewed studies to back up the claim.

A 2011 study titled "Anticancer Activities of *Nigella sativa*, Black Cumin" demonstrated potent effects against several types of cancer, including blood, lung, kidney, liver, prostate, breast, cervical, and skin.[41] The exact molecular mechanisms are still being explored, but research shows that thymoquinone may enhance the body's antioxidant defense system, promote apoptosis, which is the natural death of abnormal cells, and regulate the signaling pathways involved in cancer progression.[42] The anti-cancer effects of *Nigella sativa* have been recognized for thousands of years in traditional medicine, but modern scientific validation has emerged in just the past two to three decades. The research is growing, and the results are promising.

Black cumin seed oil is one of those supplements you absolutely want to take in capsule form. Anyone who has ever tried the straight oil will tell you that it tastes horrible. You do not want it in a smoothie, and you definitely do not want to take it by the spoonful. If you try that, you will probably be so repulsed that you will never take it again. This is why I made Hashimoto's Support by the Fixxr, which contains black cumin seed oil standardized to 3 percent of the active ingredient thymoquinone in capsule form. You get the therapeutic dose of the active compound without the taste, and you are far more likely to be consistent in taking it.

In my practice, I have seen patients achieve truly remarkable results from taking black cumin seed oil, even pushing their Hashimoto's into remission. I cannot promise that result for everyone, but when it happens, it is powerful.

Black Cumin Seed Oil Protocol

Most brands offer 500 or 1,000 mg capsules, but it's the percentage of thymoquinone in each capsule that really matters. You could be taking a 1,000 mg capsule but getting only 1 percent thymoquinone. One to two capsules, each with 3 percent thymoquinone, daily is ideal.

Hashimoto's Support by the Fixxr Protocol

Take one to two capsules per day at any time of day. Consistent use supports antibody reduction, inflammation control, and overall thyroid and immune system balance.

Selenium

Selenium plays a direct role in both the creation and the metabolism of thyroid hormones and has potent antioxidant properties that impact the thyroid gland itself. Your thyroid naturally contains selenium, and this trace mineral is essential for the function of several selenoproteins that help convert T4 to T3, protect the thyroid gland from oxidative stress, and support overall hormone balance.[43]

It makes sense, then, that selenium deficiency can lead to a variety of thyroid issues, such as Hashimoto's thyroiditis, goiter, and even hyper-thyroidism, including Graves' disease.[44] It is also one of the few nutrients shown in studies to help lower thyroid peroxidase (TPO) antibodies,[45] a key marker in thyroid autoimmune disease.

The best form of selenium to take as a supplement is selenome-thionine. This organic form has a 90 percent absorption rate and is far more effective than other forms, which do not provide the same absorption rate or targeted thyroid benefits. You can also get selenium from food. Brazil nuts, fish, and whole grains are solid sources. But let's be honest: If you are avoiding grains to reduce inflammation and you are not a fan of fish or Brazil nuts, supplementation is probably the way to go.

Be aware, however, that with selenium, more is not better. Excessive intake can be toxic, especially if you are getting it from more than source. Once you go over 400 mcg a day, you are in the danger zone. I have seen thyroid patients who read something online and started consuming a lot more selenium than they should, thinking it was a magic fix. But instead of helping, it drove up their reverse T3 and made them feel worse.

Selenium is a "Goldilocks" supplement: You want the dose to be just right, not too little, not too much, just enough to support your thyroid without tipping things in the wrong direction. My recommendation is 100 mcg per day. That is a safe and effective dose for most people. My T3 Conversion Fixxr contains 100 mcg of selenium. And when you combine it with other "No Duh" supplements, particularly conversion helpers such as magnesium and iodine, you can support your thyroid naturally, lower your reverse T3, and finally feel your body moving in the right direction.

Selenium Protocol
 Take 100 mcg per day.

T3 Conversion Fixxr Protocol
 Take one serving per day to provide 100 mcg of selenium. This supports T4 to T3 conversion, lowers inflammation, and supports immune balance in the thyroid.

Ashwagandha

Ashwagandha is an adaptogenic plant long used in Ayurvedic medicine that promotes healthy cortisol balance. The word *adaptogen* refers to plants used in herbal medicine that can help the body adapt to and resist stressors (one familiar example is ginseng). Ashwagandha is believed to reduce the amount of cortisol that your body produces, and studies have shown that it can also improve sleep, calm anxiety, and support overall resilience to stress.[46]

As we've seen, thyroid function is directly impacted by elevated cortisol. When we lower stress and keep cortisol levels down, inflammation decreases, T4 to T3 conversion improves, and hypothyroidism symptoms improve. Taking ashwagandha supports these efforts, stabilizing the physiological environment around your thyroid so it can function without constantly feeling like it is under attack.

Ashwagandha Protocol
 Take 300–600 mg per day to support cortisol balance, stress resilience, mood stability, and thyroid hormone conversion.

T3 Conversion Fixxr Protocol
 Take one serving per day to provide 200 mg of ashwagandha, balance your cortisol, and support T4 to T3 conversion.

The "No Duh" Supplements Starter Protocol

Below is what I consider to be a reasonable, effective starter protocol for optimizing thyroid health. It is safe to use alongside your thyroid medications and has scientific backing behind it. You don't need to take all these to start, and some (such as iodine) require titration over time to reach your optimal dose. If seven supplements seems overwhelming, pick one or two that seem to match your specific needs. If you want to start with only one, take iodine. If you can manage only two, add vitamin D. You can also work with a doctor to figure out what combination is best for you.

Naturally, I believe that my Fixxr supplements deliver the best results, and I take them every day myself. But you can use this protocol and the other information in this chapter to assemble your own regimen using brands of your choosing. Just be sure that you are buying *high-quality* products. If you buy a product on Amazon because it's less expensive, you likely aren't getting a supplement with the same potency or purity, which almost certainly means that you won't get the same results.

Supplement	Dosage	Purpose (in Brief)
Iodine Fixxr	Start with 1 drop per day; increase by 1 drop per day until you reach 6–50 mg.	Supports thyroid hormone production, metabolism, and overall energy.
Quad Magnesium by the Fixxr	Take 2 capsules at night (or in the daytime if preferred).	Improves sleep, calms the nervous system, reduces stress.
Vit D Fixxr	Take 1 capsule daily, with dietary fat.	Supports thyroid hormone function, immunity, mood, and calcium utilization.
B Fixxr	Take 1 serving per day.	Supports thyroid hormone production, energy, methylation, and neurotransmitters.
Hashimoto's Support by the Fixxr (black cumin seed oil)	Take 1–2 capsules per day.	Helps calm inflammation and support reduction of thyroid antibodies.
T3 Conversion Fixxr (selenium and ashwagangha)	Take 1 serving per day.	Supports T4 to T3 conversion, lowers inflammation, supports immunity, balances cortisol, and improves stress resilience.

Additional Supplement Support

I want to mention a few other supplements that I consider optional but potentially helpful. This is where things get more personalized. These are not your daily "No Duh" supplements, but they can be health changers when used correctly and under the guidance of a practitioner who knows what they are doing:

Berberine

Berberine has been shown to help with glucose control, improve insulin sensitivity, and support weight loss, all areas that thyroid patients struggle with.[47] I use berberine supplements with patients in a targeted way to address insulin resistance. 1,200 mg per day is the therapeutic dose, which is why my Blood Sugar Fixxr contains 600 mg of berberine per capsule. Take one capsule with each of your main or largest meals. Ideally, you should take it before a meal so it can help control your glucose and insulin response to that meal. But if you forget, taking it with or shortly after a meal is still effective.

Tongkat Ali and *Tribulus terrestris*

In my clinic we use testosterone-supporting supplements such as tongkat ali and *Tribulus terrestris*, which is included in my Hormone Fixxr, to boost a woman's testosterone naturally. Tongkat ali, in particular, is believed to increase your free testosterone by lowering your level of sex hormone–binding globulin (SHBG).[48] We use bioidentical testosterone replacement as well, often alongside Hormone Fixxr. Testosterone is incredibly protective against autoimmunity, inflammation, and even mood and muscle loss. In contrast, low testosterone can worsen autoimmune symptoms and lead to rising antibody levels.

Unfortunately, it is difficult for most women to find a doctor who understands the benefits of testosterone for thyropause and menopause, so they must try to boost their level naturally through supplementation. I have also found that even if you are on testosterone therapy, Hormone Fixxr gives a lift to your results at the gym. I am always just a little bit stronger and my muscles look better when I take Hormone Fixxr alongside testosterone.

Melatonin

If you are not sleeping well due to inflammation or poorly regulated blood sugar, hormones, or adrenals, these symptoms all lead back to your thyroid. Melatonin is a sleep aid with antiviral properties that supports the immune system by activating natural killer cell pathways. That means it can help with viral load and even provide some protection against cancer.[49] Most important, it can help you get the deep, restorative sleep your body needs to heal.

Creatine

Creatine is often marketed to male bodybuilders, but it is one of the most underrated supplements for women, especially those in perimenopause and menopause. Creatine supports ATP production in your muscles and brain, which means better strength, power, and cognitive function.[50] As estrogen and progesterone decline, many women notice that they have more brain fog, slower muscle recovery, and a harder time building or maintaining muscle in general. Creatine helps offset these changes by supporting muscle performance and protecting brain health. For thyroid patients who are already fighting fatigue and muscle weakness, creatine can be a simple addition that makes workouts feel more productive and mental tasks a little easier.

Digestive Enzymes

Many Hashimoto's patients are low in stomach acid, which leads to bloating, indigestion, and slow digestion. My Digest Fixxr supplies both digestive enzymes and betaine hydrochloride (similar to the hydrochloric acid found in your stomach) so that you can properly absorb nutrients and support your overall metabolic health. Taking one to two capsules with meals helps reduce bloating, improves digestion, facilitates the proper breakdown of protein, fats, and carbohydrates, and promotes better nutrient absorption.

Liver Fixxr

Your liver plays a major role in T4 to T3 conversion, but it also serves as your body's epicenter for detoxification. When your liver is sluggish and overburdened, T4 conversion slows and your symptoms worsen. My Liver Fixxr supports detox pathways, efficient T3 production, and the breakdown and clearance of excess hormones (such as cortisol), all of which are vital when you are trying to optimize your thyroid function. Its primary ingredient, milk thistle, has been shown to lower inflammation in the liver,[51] which ensures that your liver can efficiently carry out its many jobs.

• • •

I could list dozens of other supportive supplements that work for specific scenarios or symptom clusters. Beyond my starter protocol, your best approach is to work with someone who understands the thyroid inside and out and build a supplement protocol that fits your body's and your own needs.

Always remember that supplements are meant to support your thyroid and hormones, not replace the core treatments you need. When used strategically, they can enhance your body's natural pathways and help your thyroid function at a higher level. Your job now is to understand what each product in your routine is trying to address and to be honest about what is working and what is not. Start with the "No Duh" list, add a few targeted supports if you truly need them, and let the rest go. That is how you build a supplement plan that will actually support your thyroid and your life, instead of running it.

If You Could Take Only One Supplement to Support Your Thyroid . . .

If I could take only *one* supplement every day to support my health and thyroid, it would be nascent iodine. So this is where I say: If you are wary of supplements, if you think they're too expensive, or if you just want to keep things simple—take iodine. I give you permission to skip everything else. My hope is that you'll add others down the line, because I know how they can enhance your progress and I know how much better they can make you feel. But if you want to start simple, start here.

If I could take only *two* supplements, they would be nascent iodine and vitamin D3. This powerful duo packs a punch and does wonders for your thyroid and your body as a whole. Adding other supplements will build on their benefits, but taking one or two is far better than taking none at all.

Chapter 10

T2: The Forgotten Thyroid Hormone

I still remember the frustration I used to feel before my clinic could prescribe in all fifty states. I'd be consulting with patients whose doctors had them stuck on T4-only medication year after year, and they were miserable. They were gaining weight, exhausted, foggy, and losing hope. I knew they needed something more, something to move the needle and give them back their lives, but I didn't have the authority to change their prescriptions.

I wanted to do more, so I started digging deeper into the research on 3,5-diiodo-L-thyronine, the "other thyroid hormone," also known as T2. Fifteen years ago, hardly anyone was talking about it. It was this overlooked hormone hiding in plain sight, and the science around it, as I soon discovered, was fascinating. T2 is produced by the thyroid gland as one of the four thyroid hormones and is also created when your body metabolizes T3. It directly stimulates mitochondrial activity, and it has a significant impact on fat burning and energy.[1] If it truly worked in the ways the science was suggesting, I thought it could change everything for my patients.

I'll never forget my patient Leslie, one of the first women to whom I recommended T2. She was in her forties, had been stuck on T4 only for years, and no matter what she did, the scale kept creeping up. She was doing everything "right": eating clean, exercising, taking her meds, yet she still felt as though she was dragging her body through quicksand. When she started taking T2, the change was almost immediate.

Her energy picked up, her clothes started fitting better, and within a few months she was down twenty pounds. But more than that, she felt alive again. She told me, "For the first time in years, I feel like myself."

That's why I was so excited to write this chapter, because T2 truly is the forgotten hormone that everyone needs to know about. It has the potential to be the next big thing in the fight against obesity and fatigue because of the way it can transform metabolism, body composition, and energy. Imagine being able to burn fat while simply sitting around and having steady, reliable energy all day long, better insulin sensitivity, and the kind of cardiovascular benefits that you get from exercising—without ever hitting the gym. That's the power of T2.

What Is T2?

T2, or 3,5 diiodo-l-thyronine, is created when your body breaks down other thyroid hormones, most notably T3. Think of it this way: Your thyroid makes T4 and T3, and once T3 has done its job in a particular cell, your body processes it further, creating metabolites. Metabolites are chemical substances that are used or produced during the process of metabolism, and while some of them are inactive leftovers, others are biologically active and still have important work to do. T2 is one of those active metabolites.

What makes T2 so exciting is that it is active from the get-go (unlike T4, which needs to be converted to become active). It acts directly on your cells' mitochondria, the powerhouses of the cell where energy is produced, to increase cellular respiration and boost the production of ATP. By improving your mitochondrial efficiency, T2 increases the amount of energy you burn at rest, enhances fat oxidation (the converting of fat cells into energy), and supports healthy metabolic function overall without overstimulating your nervous system. Thus it is a potent modulator of metabolism that has a major impact on how your body uses and burns fuel.

Research has been done on T2 for more than thirty years, and the findings show that it can do things that no other thyroid hormone or fat burner can do. It can increase your resting metabolic rate without raising your heart rate or blood pressure, lower your triglyceride and cholesterol levels, and even influence your gene expression to reduce fat accumulation.[2] And unlike many stimulants or "quick fix" weight loss products, it achieves these results without spiking your cortisol, wrecking your adrenals, or disrupting your thyroid labs.

In other words, T2 is your thyroid's secret weapon to fire up your metabolism, and your body already knows how to use it. But when thyroid function is low, T2 is underproduced. By replacing it in the right amount, you can restore a missing piece of your metabolic puzzle.

What the Studies Show

I believe that T2 is one of the most exciting tools we have right now for increasing metabolism and fat loss. We are also learning that it does far more than boost your calorie burn. Recent research shows that it can turn on a gene that prevents fat accumulation.[3] Let that sink in for a moment. We are talking about flipping a genetic switch that stops your body from laying down massive amounts of fat. For years, we thought that our genes were a fixed blueprint, but now we have proof that we can potentially influence them in ways that will change how our body stores fat. That is groundbreaking.

T2 has also been shown to lower inflammation and oxidative stress,[4] both of which can wreak havoc on your metabolism, thyroid, and overall health. Less inflammation means better cellular communication. Less oxidative stress means less cellular damage. Together, that creates a healthier, more efficient environment for your thyroid and every other organ and system in your body to do their job.

These results have been shown to be true in humans as well as lab animals, and we have the studies to back it up. One human study done in 2011 looked at T2 administration to see how it impacted metabolism and fat loss.[5] The researchers studied only two people, but the testing was meticulous. They measured body weight, BMI, blood pressure, and heart rate, and did electrocardiograms, thyroid and liver ultrasounds, and testing to track cholesterol, triglyceride, free T3, free T4, T2, and TSH levels, as well as resting metabolic rate. All those were measured before treatment with T2 and again afterward. The results were incredible: After three weeks of the participants' taking 300 mcg of T2 per day, their resting metabolic rate had increased and their body fat percentage had dropped by 4 percent, amounting to a weight loss of nearly nine pounds. There were no changes in their free T3, free T4, or TSH and no cardiac side effects. In other words, their thyroid labs stayed stable and their hearts remained healthy.

To put this into perspective, an increase in resting metabolic rate and a 4 percent reduction in body fat percentage is considerable. It means that the study participants were burning more calories every day without lifting a finger, just by living their lives. And they lost substantial weight without changing their diet, without stimulants, and without that over-caffeinated, heart-racing feeling you get from sketchy fat burners.

Researchers have gone even deeper in animal studies. In one study in 2019,[6] rats were deliberately overfed a high-fat diet designed to make them obese. This was not a gentle "cheat meal" situation; it was a deliberate plan to pack on as much body fat as possible. T2 worked in this scenario, too. Notably, it converted portions of the rats' white fat to brown fat, increased their thermogenesis, and pulled stored fat right off them.

I've talked about white and brown fat before. White fat is the storage fat that most of us think of, the kind that pads the belly, hips, and thighs while holding on to energy for "later" (which, let's be honest, never seems to come). Brown fat, however, is metabolically active. Instead of hoarding energy, it burns calories to generate heat, and it is loaded with mitochondria. These extra, iron-rich mitochondria are what give brown fat its reddish brown color. When T2 "browns" white fat, it is spurring the creation of additional mitochondria, essentially upgrading useless storage fat into fat that burns calories and produces energy. That is like converting your old, dusty garage into a high-performance engine room. More brown fat means more built-in calorie burn, even when you are at rest.

Whether you are eating low carb, high carb, high fat, or somewhere in between, none of that changes the basic law of energy balance: If you consistently take in more energy than you burn, your body will store it. Your metabolism has the ability to adapt somewhat, but if you are consistently eating a surplus, you will still gain fat. What is remarkable in this study is that even when the animals were intentionally overfed—in other words, when the deck was stacked against them—T2 still shifted the needle toward fat burning, metabolic activity, and better overall energy balance.

One fascinating 2021 finding among the various studies showed that T2 activated brown adipose tissue thermogenesis in hypothyroid rats.[7] The rats already had slower metabolisms because they were hypothyroid, and it is not as though they were optimized on medication, eating clean, or exercising. Yet even in a low metabolic state, T2 triggered fat loss and reduced the rats' fat mass.

Even more amazing, T2 does all this without impacting the overall function of the thyroid gland. Multiple animal studies showed no impact on free T3, free T4, or TSH. Even when the animals were deliberately overfed, T2 prevented fatty liver disease, improved their insulin sensitivity, lowered their cholesterol levels, and kept their body weight from climbing.[8]

Unlocking the Potential of T2

When I first started exploring T2, I wanted to test it in real life, outside the lab, with real women having real struggles. I brought together eleven women ages twenty-eight to sixty-five, all with different body types and backgrounds. Some had only ten pounds to lose; others had fifty or more. Some had hypothyroidism, some didn't. A few were menopausal and not on any hormones at all.

And here's an important point: We didn't intervene as if they were my patients in any other respect. We didn't optimize their thyroid meds, we didn't put them on hormones, we didn't change anything about their treatment. All we did was put them on Thyroid Fixxr, or Metabolism

Fixxr®, both of which contain 150 mcg of T2, to see how their bodies would respond.

The results blew us away. Every single woman lost weight. In just sixteen weeks, they dropped between fifteen and forty-five pounds each. Those who weren't being treated properly for their thyroid dysfunction, the T4-only women, still lost weight. Those with no hormones on board at all dropped at least ten pounds. It was an indication that T2 could shift metabolism regardless of baseline.

Michelle was one of those women. She had just come out of cancer treatment and was still on prednisone, a drug that makes fat loss nearly impossible. She didn't expect much to happen when she started T2; she figured maybe she'd feel a little better, but she wasn't holding her breath. Sixteen weeks later, the scale told a different story: She was down an astonishing forty pounds. For the first time since her cancer diagnosis, she felt that she had control over her body again instead of feeling as though the disease and its medications had taken everything from her.

Then there was Rachel, a twenty-nine-year-old nurse. She'd had thyroid problems since her teens but had never gotten proper treatment. She pushed herself through long hospital shifts, exhausted and carrying stubborn weight she couldn't shake no matter what diet, workout, or trick she tried. After sixteen weeks on T2, she finally dropped the weight that had haunted her for over a decade. More important, she told me she could finally keep up with her patients and her life again without running on fumes.

Anna was a forty-two-year-old mother of three. She was dragging herself through every day, so tired that guilt became her constant companion. "I feel like a bad mom," she admitted, "because I don't even have the energy to play with my kids." The extra weight made her feel heavy in every way — not just physically but emotionally. It was stealing her joy. On T2, she lost twenty-five pounds, her energy came back, and she told me she finally felt present with her kids again.

Incredibly, T2 burns fat and improves energy even when the odds are stacked against you. Reading about the science is one thing, but when you see it come alive in real women, the results are undeniable.

One thing I want to emphasize, however, is that T2 is *not* a substitute for T3. T2 works wonders for energy and metabolism, but it cannot supply the T3 hormone that every cell in your body needs for brain function, sleep, reproductive health, digestive health, and all the rest. T2 should be viewed as an add-on bonus to thoughtful, personalized prescription hormone treatment. If you have hypothyroidism, you can't be truly optimized and feel your best without T3, and often without T4.

Burn Fat, Not Muscle: The Bodybuilder Backstory

One of the most incredible features of T2 is that it targets fat but doesn't burn muscle. As any exercise physiologist, weight loss expert, or prescriber of GLP-1s will tell you, it's not always easy to achieve significant weight loss without cannibalizing muscle.

Historically, bodybuilders and fitness athletes have used thyroid hormones off-label to keep their body fat percentage down. Bodybuilders were the original biohackers. They were experimenting with peptides, selective androgen receptor modulators (SARMs), cold plunges, and other cutting-edge hacks before the general public had ever heard of them. In particular, they were using T3 obtained on the black market without a prescription to strip away body fat. When you take thyroid medication and don't have a thyroid problem, it creates a negative feedback loop that shuts down your own hormone production. In someone who is already hypothyroid, we are replacing what is missing. But in a healthy person, you are risking permanent hypothyroidism. And because T3 burns both fat and muscle, it can leave you smaller but not necessarily leaner or healthier.

I once watched an interview with one of the top trainers in professional bodybuilding and figure competition, a guy who had worked with some of the best athletes in the world, the ones who live or die by how much muscle they keep while stripping away every ounce of fat before they step onstage. What he said confirmed what I had been seeing in my own patients for years: He said that he absolutely refused to let his athletes use T3. Sure, T3 would peel fat off the body, but at a cost: It would chew up muscle and could wreck the thyroid. In the world of bodybuilding, muscle is everything. You don't sacrifice it. And once you suppress your thyroid function, it's a long, hard road to get it back.

What that trainer did use instead was T2. He had found what I'd been seeing: T2 burned only fat. It preserved lean muscle. It didn't overstimulate the heart or jack up blood pressure. And when the contest prep was over, his athletes' thyroids bounced back. No lingering dysfunction, no permanent damage. Hearing him say that was so validating, because it echoed what I'd been watching unfold in real people in my practice. My patients on T2 were burning fat, holding on to their muscle, and not wrecking their thyroids in the process.

T2 is an exercise mimetic in that it gives you the same mitochondrial benefits as exercise does. No, you can't just sit on the couch and wait for miracles to happen. But if you combine T2 with movement, training, and the other good things you're already doing, you get a multiplier effect. It stacks right on top of your efforts, making everything you're doing fitnesswise work even better. We know that exercise improves insulin sensitivity, lowers leptin, reduces body fat, increases thermogenesis, improves cholesterol, and supports liver health. It turns out that T2 does all that, too.

Protecting Your Thyroid with T2

When your thyroid produces thyroid hormone, free radicals are created as part of the process. That's normal. What's not normal is when your thyroid does not have enough antioxidant protection to neutralize those free radicals. This leaves the gland vulnerable to oxidative stress, and oxidative stress is one of the biggest drivers of thyroid dysfunction.

Glutathione is your body's master antioxidant. It is produced in the liver, and its job is to neutralize free radicals, clear toxins, support detox pathways, and keep your mitochondria working efficiently. When glutathione is low, oxidative stress builds up,[9] and that's like rust slowly wearing down the machinery of your thyroid cells. Over time this damage can trigger autoimmune activity, worsen Hashimoto's, impair thyroid hormone conversion, and keep your metabolism sluggish no matter what medication you are on.

This is why combining T2 with glutathione makes sense. T2 supports mitochondrial function and metabolic activity, while glutathione provides antioxidant protection that helps lower the oxidative stress interfering with thyroid hormone action. Together they support the two areas in which most thyroid patients struggle: low mitochondrial output and high inflammation. This is exactly why we formulated my T2 cream with glutathione. Applying it directly over the thyroid gives you both the metabolic support of T2 and the antioxidant protection of glutathione right where your body needs it most.

In addition to topical application, glutathione can be taken as a supplement, but how you take it matters. It is best absorbed as a sublingual liposomal formula or through an IV. Oral capsules are not recommended because they must pass through the digestive tract, which breaks them down and significantly limits absorption. If you are going to supplement glutathione, choose a form your body can actually use.

One of my patients had been struggling for years with weight gain, swelling, fatigue, and brain fog, even though she was already on thyroid medication. Her provider had kept telling her that everything was fine. She had tried various diets with zero success. Within a few weeks of using the T2 and glutathione cream, she said it felt as though her whole system was finally unclogged. Her afternoon crashes disappeared, her face and hands lost their inflamed puffiness, and her mental clarity started coming back. Over the next three months, she dropped eighteen pounds without extreme dieting, and her antibody levels began to improve. She said, "It feels like someone turned the lights back on in my body."

That's the impact of T2 when it is paired with glutathione. It is not just about losing weight; it is about lowering the oxidative stress that has been holding your thyroid function back, restoring energy you thought was gone for good, and finally giving your metabolism the support it needed all along.

No Prescription Needed

The best part of all this is that T2 is available over the counter. That's right. Something this powerful, and you don't have to beg your doctor for a prescription. You don't have to sit in another exam room, explaining your symptoms for the tenth time, only to be handed an antidepressant or told to "eat less, move more." T2 bypasses all that. It doesn't alter your thyroid labs or overstimulate your heart, and it doesn't carry the risks of so many weight loss "quick fixes." It's safe, effective, and accessible. Whether you've been diagnosed with a thyroid condition or not, your metabolism can benefit from T2.

When I first started using T2 with my patients about fifteen years ago, the only option on the market came in one of those hardcore "bro science" power-lifting formulas. You know what I mean: It came in a huge black tub with a giant flexing gorilla plastered across the label. Picture me telling a forty-five-year-old perimenopausal woman who was already skeptical, "Don't worry, this will help your thyroid and metabolism. Just go buy the one with the gorilla." You can imagine the look I got. Not exactly a match made in Heaven.

That experience stuck with me. When I created my supplement line, I knew T2 had to be front and center, and I developed a clean, trusted, effective product that made sense for women. My Thyroid Fixxr formula is built around T2 but paired with additional ingredients that support metabolism and thyroid function, including L-tyrosine, the amino acid your thyroid uses to produce thyroid hormone. Unlike a lot of the "bro" formulas on the market, which contain a bunch of what I consider to be unnecessary ingredients such as caffeine, T2 is the focus of my formula. We believe that 150 mcg of T2 is all you need to see results.

Of course, the inevitable question comes up: "Can I take this if I don't have a thyroid issue?" The answer is absolutely. The name of certain products might make you think otherwise, but you don't need to have a thyroid problem to reap the benefits. That's why I also created Metabolism Fixxr with the same dose of T2 but branded clearly so that anyone looking to boost their energy, improve their insulin sensitivity, and rev up their fat loss can feel confident using it.

If you're sitting there wondering whether T2 could be the missing piece in your puzzle, the answer is probably yes. If you want to have steady energy, a sharper metabolism, and fat loss without sacrificing your thyroid or your muscle, this is it. This is the tool I had been waiting for, and now it's the tool you've been waiting for, too.

Chapter 11

Eat This, Not That

If you have a thyroid problem, what you eat is working either for you or against you. There's no middle ground. You can't keep eating like everyone else does and expect to heal. Your thyroid, immune system, and metabolism are directly impacted by what you put into your body. But I also said from the very beginning that this is not a diet book, and I've never claimed that simply eating certain foods would magically fix your thyroid. Food alone doesn't heal a broken thyroid, and no perfect diet can override poor thyroid function. At the same time, if you're constantly putting garbage into your body, there's no amount of thyroid medication that can extinguish the internal dumpster fire that creates.

And the flip side matters just as much. You can find the diet that feels perfect for you, the one where you're eating clean, hitting your protein, doing everything right, and if your thyroid is still in the toilet, that diet is eventually going to stop working, too. That's when Screw It Syndrome shows up. Screw It Syndrome is what happens when you are eating perfectly, nothing is working, you don't feel better, the scale keeps going up, and by the end of the day you just say, "Screw it," and eat the pizza and cookies because it feels like nothing makes a difference anymore.

I know that some of you will hate hearing this. We all want choosing our food to be simple, and I'm not here to make it complicated. But if you really want to feel better, this is one of the strongest levers you can pull. Food isn't the be-all and end-all, but it absolutely plays a role. In this chapter, I'll give you straight-up guidance about which diets tend to work best to support thyroid health, along with my honest take on some of the biggest hot-button foods and trends, starting with everyone's favorite dietary villain: gluten.

Gluten

Going gluten free isn't a trend or an optional checkbox, it's a biochemical must. If you have any level of thyroid dysfunction, especially Hashimoto's, going gluten free isn't about being "cruel" to carbs. It's about protecting your thyroid from your own immune system.

Gluten, a structural protein complex found in grains such as wheat, barley, and rye, contains a protein called gliadin, which your immune system tags as a threat. This happens in all of us, regardless of whether you experience any sort of reaction or digestive discomfort when you eat gluten. As luck would have it, gliadin and your thyroid tissue look alarmingly similar. This is called *molecular mimicry*. When you eat gluten, your immune system gears up to attack gliadin, but it ends up attacking your thyroid by mistake.[1] This leads to more inflammation, more antibodies, and more damage to a thyroid gland that is already struggling. Gliadin also triggers the release of zonulin, a protein that opens junctions between the cells in the gut, making it more permeable to foreign organisms and toxins. When the gut becomes more permeable, immune system activation rises, which increases total-body inflammation and fuels autoimmunity.

I always hear, "But I don't feel anything when I eat bread." I get it. You may not have an immediate, discernable reaction, but that doesn't mean that the damage isn't happening under the surface. Both TPO antibodies and TgAb can spike for up to six months from just one exposure. I love this saying: "Being kind of gluten-free is like being kind of pregnant." It's impossible. One bite is still enough to trigger your immune system.

People who are strictly and truly 100 percent gluten free know this firsthand. Their systems are so clear that when gluten sneaks in at a restaurant or in a mislabeled food, their body reacts right away. It might be bloating, stomach pain, migraines, joint pain, or even sudden weight gain. That's why you'll hear them say "I've been glutened." They feel it because their body is no longer inflamed all the time, so the reaction is obvious when it happens.

When you first make the shift to being fully gluten free, it can be intimidating. I know what you're thinking; you're questioning whether you will ever be able to eat and enjoy the foods you love again, and you're worrying that everything gluten free is going to taste awful. Just trust me on this one . . . once you get into it and begin experimenting with various gluten-free swaps, you'll realize that it's not only doable, it's enjoyable! Because P.S., some foods actually taste better in their gluten-free form. I am not saying you should binge on gluten-free pretzels, but OMG, they are kind of the bomb.

If you need a little more incentive to try a gluten-free lifestyle, here's what you can expect to notice pretty quickly after cutting gluten: Bloating eases, your stomach calms down, your joints stop screaming, your brain clears, and believe it or not, those random headaches or migraines you've always had start to disappear. Many people also notice that they have steadier energy, fewer cravings, and an easier time losing weight simply because the hidden inflammation is no longer there. But the biggest benefit by far is that you're no longer aiding and abetting the attack and destruction of your thyroid gland.

When you go gluten free, the beginning is always the hardest part. Just hang in there. Once you get comfortable in the kitchen again, you'll discover recipes and products that taste amazing, and you really will stop missing gluten. There are countless gluten-free cookbooks, food bloggers, and recipe sites to make the transition simple. And you can always just ask Alexa to find you a gluten-free recipe for anything.

One more point that needs to be made: Going gluten free doesn't mean buying everything that has "gluten free" stamped on the label. That's one of the largest traps out there. Years ago, you couldn't find anything gluten free. If you wanted crackers, you were in your kitchen making them yourself from scratch with almond flour. Now entire aisles of gluten-free snacks and breads populate grocery stores. However, you should know that a lot of those products are loaded with sugar and filled with inflammatory grains that are just as bad for you as gluten. We'll delve into those grains in the next section, because they deserve their own spotlight.

Grains

Even if you've cut out gluten, other grains can still trip you up. Just because a product is labeled "gluten free" doesn't mean it's safe. Corn, rice, oats, and quinoa can all make your gut leakier and increase inflammation. Most grains today are sprayed with glyphosate, the pesticide I talked about in chapter 3 that is a known endocrine disruptor. It messes with your hormones and tears up your gut lining.[2]

Recall that about 20 percent of your T4 to T3 conversion happens in the gut. If your gut is inflamed or your microbiome is off, you're not going to convert well. Some people can bring back small amounts of gluten-free grains into their diet once their gut is healed and their immune system calms down. But in the beginning, especially if you have active autoimmunity, you need to be strict. Think of it as giving both your gut and your thyroid a reset.

This doesn't mean you're left with nothing to eat. Swap rice for cauliflower rice. Bake with almond, coconut, or cassava flour. Skip oats and try chia pudding or hemp hearts. For crunchy snacks, go with flax crackers or almond flour crackers. Opt for spaghetti squash or zucchini noodles instead of pasta. Again, ask Alexa to find whatever recipe your heart desires. If you want to go old school, go to any local bookstore and hit the food section. There are plenty of gluten-free cookbooks. I tend to recommend paleo gluten-free recipes because they focus on good-quality protein and healthy fats and eliminate all processed foods. Look for the book *Against All Grain: Delectable Paleo Recipes to Eat Well & Feel Great* by Danielle Walker, or grab the *How Can It Be Gluten Free Cookbook Collection* by America's Test Kitchen for your home cooking enjoyment.

Dairy Products

This one is personal. Some people react strongly to dairy products, often because of proteins such as casein. For them, dairy products can trigger bloating, sinus congestion, stomach upset, or skin issues. I've had patients tell me for years, "Oh, dairy doesn't bother me," only to realize once they cut it out that the nagging skin breakouts, constant sinus pressure, and afternoon bloat they thought was "normal" were tied to their consumption of cheese or cream.

Not everyone reacts that way. Some people tolerate dairy products just fine, especially when they're high quality. I'm one of them. I consume grass-fed cheeses, Kerrygold butter, and organic half-and-half in my coffee. I don't overdo them, but I don't avoid them, either, because they don't give me trouble.

The best way to know if you are sensitive to dairy products is to test yourself. Leave them out of your diet for a few weeks, then add them back in and pay close attention to how your gut feels, whether your skin breaks out, if your sinuses flare up, or if your energy level shifts. Your body will tell you quickly whether dairy products are friends or foes.

If it turns out that your body says no, you're not stuck. There are plenty of clean alternatives. Ghee is a great butter substitute because the milk proteins are almost entirely removed. For coffee, try unsweetened almond or coconut milk. If you like yogurt, there are good versions made from coconut, almond, or cashew. Even cheeses now exist that are made from cashews or almonds, and some of them are pretty convincing. It takes some experimenting, but once you find what works for you, it's easier than you think to live without traditional dairy products.

Protein

Protein becomes more important as we age. I know that might surprise you because you probably look at your grandparents picking at half a sandwich and think, "I could eat three of those and still be hungry." Our appetite does decrease as we get older because we aren't as active as we were in our twenties, so it's easy to assume that we don't need as much food. What we do need more of, however, is protein.

As we age, our bodies naturally start losing muscle, a process called *sarcopenia*. Less muscle means less support for your bones, a weaker body, a slower metabolism, more fat gain, and a much higher risk of falls and injuries because your overall physical structure is less stable. Protein is what fights back. It gives your body the raw materials to build lean, strong muscle tissue. When you eat good bioavailable protein, such as eggs, fish, chicken, beef, or collagen, you give your body the amino acids it needs to repair and build muscle. That's what keeps you strong. That's what keeps your metabolism running instead of slowing down with age.

Protein also stimulates the production of a hormone called insulin-like growth factor (IGF-1).[3] IGF-1 is connected to human growth hormone (HGH), another hormone that declines as we age. HGH is the "upstream" hormone that signals to your liver to produce IGF-1, which then acts on cells throughout the body to protect your muscles, keep your skin plump, hold back wrinkles, and keep your body in a more youthful state. It naturally drops starting around age thirty, which is why our energy, skin, and muscle tone all take a hit. By eating enough protein, you can bump up your IGF-1 level, which means nudging your overall level of growth hormone in the right direction. Anytime you can do that naturally, it's a win.

Even if you feel like eating less as the years go by, protein is the one thing you can't cut back on. If you don't have the appetite for a twelve-ounce grass-fed rib-eye steak, keep it simple: Blend a high-quality beef isolate protein with ice and almond milk and drink it like a milkshake. Get jiggy with it by adding berries, a scoop of almond butter, even cacao powder for a rich chocolate flavor. And don't be afraid to double up on the scoops if you're not eating much whole food protein. Yes, I'm talking to *you*, ladies!

The bonus here is that protein is incredibly satiating. It curbs your hunger, helps you feel satisfied and full, won't spike your blood sugar, and reduces the temptation to snack on processed junk. Protein consumption quiets the "food noise" you may be experiencing.

Protein can even help with some classic hypothyroid symptoms, such as dry skin, brittle nails, and hair that sheds or feels like straw. Your hair is built from a protein called keratin, and your body needs amino acids from protein to make it. Same with your nails: If you're not getting enough protein, your body doesn't have the building blocks to keep your hair thick and your nails strong.

I recommend aiming for 1 gram of protein per pound of your ideal body weight or lean body mass. If your happy weight is 150 pounds, aim for 150 grams of protein per day. If you're a woman and your ideal weight is 180 pounds, you might find that 180 grams feels like too much food. In that case, start with 130 to 140 grams, monitor how you feel, and increase gradually.

I'll pause here to point out that while some in the medical community have raised the alarm about too much protein in recent years—with some headlines even suggesting that it can be toxic—I completely disagree with the idea that high protein intake can be harmful. In fact, all the research I've seen suggests that higher protein intake is not only safe for healthy individuals, it is protective and foundational for long-term health. Protein provides the raw materials your body needs to build and repair your muscles, organs, skin, enzymes, and even your DNA, which becomes increasingly important as we age.[4] Adequate protein also helps preserve lean muscle mass, prevent sarcopenia,[5] and maintain strength and physical function,[6] which directly impacts mobility, independence, and metabolic health. Higher protein intake also supports a higher resting metabolic rate,[7] improves satiety, reduces cravings, and helps preserve lean muscle during calorie restriction, which is critical for sustainable fat loss. On top of all that, the amino acids we get from protein are involved in immune function, hormone production, and energy generation, supporting ATP production and overall metabolic resilience.

When you look at the full body of evidence, protein is not the villain it is sometimes made out to be—it is one of the most powerful tools we have to support metabolism, aging, recovery, and overall health. Many leaders in the functional medicine community, including Dr. Gabrielle Lyon and JJ Virgin, consistently speak about how protein protects muscle, the organ of longevity, and how we need to eat more of it, not less, as we get older.

But let's be honest. Getting 130 to 140 grams of protein or more every day from whole foods alone is not easy. This is where a high-quality protein powder is your secret weapon. It's one of the simplest ways to increase your intake without spending your whole day chewing on chicken breast. By using a protein powder that agrees with your body, you can hit your target without feeling like it's a chore.

Let's break down the protein powder options.

The first type is the ever-popular whey protein. It was one of the first protein powders to hit the market and took off in the bodybuilding community because it was cheap and those using it could easily hit their protein targets. But whey was never designed for the average woman to drink all day. For many people, whey destroys the gut, causes bloating, disrupts digestion, and spikes insulin. Bodybuilders want that insulin spike after a workout to pump nutrients into their muscles, but a forty-five-year-old soccer mom driving to work doesn't need an insulin surge every morning.

Plant-based proteins have their own challenges. I went through a plant-based protein phase myself, thinking I was doing something good, and all I got in return was embarrassing digestive distress. As soon as I cut out the pea protein, my stomach stopped grumbling like an old radiator.

My favorite protein source is beef isolate– or beef collagen–based protein powder, which gives you all the essential amino acids in a complete source of protein without the digestive drama. The trick is finding one that doesn't taste as though you're drinking a cow.

Here's where I'm going to give a shameless plug and pat myself on the back for creating Power Protein Fixxr, because it tastes absolutely freaking amazing. It blends perfectly into a milkshake consistency, and I can drink it every day. I throw two scoops into a shake with ice and almond milk in the morning, which gives me 42 grams of protein before I've even started my day. Sometimes I'll end my day with another shake, bringing me to 84 grams of pure, clean protein without even thinking about it. Then all I have to do is eat some real food protein at lunch and dinner, and I've hit my target.

Fats

If you grew up in the 1970s or '80s, you probably still have that little voice in your head telling you that fat is the enemy. Remember the fat-free craze? That was fun. We all gained weight eating fat-free, high-sugar everything. Fat-free brownies? Heck, yes, I'll take two, they're fat free. SnackWell's cookies? A daily habit. They were fat free, so that meant they were safe, right? I can't even tell you how much weight I gained eating white rice with milk, cinnamon, and sugar in the name of being "fat free."

If you're still stuck in that mindset, it's time to break out of it. Your body needs fat—the right kind of fat. Every cell in your body has a membrane made of fat. Without it, your cells can't function. Fats also help you absorb the fat-soluble vitamins A, D, E, and K, all of which are critical for maintaining your immune system and hormone levels and reducing inflammation.

Don't fear fats; just choose the good ones. Think of avocados, wild-caught fish, grass-fed beef, olive oil, coconut oil, and pasture-raised eggs. And don't forget cholesterol. It's been demonized for decades, but it is the backbone of your hormones. Without it, your body can't make estrogen, progesterone, or testosterone in the amounts you need. No wonder so many of us who lived through the fat-free craze ended up with hormone chaos.

There is currently quite a debate around seed oils, such as canola, sunflower, corn, and grapeseed. Some experts swear they're harmless, others call them toxic. Although this statement is going to be inflammatory (pun absolutely intended), I'll say this: Avoid them when you can. They're heavily processed, are prone to oxidation, and can stir up inflammation. But don't beat yourself up if you cave and have some bar fries cooked in week-old canola oil every once in a while. It happens. The goal is progress, not perfection.

Above all, when you look at your plate, don't shy away from fat. Drizzle olive oil over your veggies, add avocado to your salad, and cook your eggs in butter or coconut oil. Fats aren't the enemy; rather, they are what your thyroid, your hormones, and your entire body need to function.

Making Dietary Changes: The 80/20 Rule, Part 2

The 80/20 rule gives some leeway in case you're sitting there thinking "Oh, my goodness, I have to completely overhaul my diet." You don't. If you can eat clean 80 percent of the time and let yourself live life the other 20 percent, you're going to be way ahead of the game. That means that most of the time you're sticking with real food, high-quality protein, healthy fats, and vegetables, and cutting out the processed junk, sugar, and seed oils. The other 20 percent is where you have the cake at your kid's birthday, enjoy a cocktail on vacation, or split the fries when you're out with friends.

The one big exception here is gluten. The 80/20 rule does not apply to gluten if you have thyroid autoimmunity problems. Even a small amount of gluten can keep your immune system attacking your thyroid for months, so that's the one thing that really has to go. With everything else, though—sugar, alcohol, seed oils, processed snacks—the 80/20 rule lets you find balance without guilt. If 80 percent of the time you're feeding your thyroid what it needs, the other 20 percent isn't going to derail you.

As you go through your day, think about the small choices you make stacking up in your favor. Every meal is a chance to either fuel inflammation or fight it. When you hit 80 percent most of the time, you'll start to notice the difference: less brain fog, more energy, less inflammation, and a body that feels as though it's finally on your side again.

You deserve to feel clear, light, and strong, and it all starts with giving your body the raw materials it needs. When you eat like your thyroid matters, everything else starts to fall into place.

Different Diets: The Pros, the Cons, and What Really Works

So many diets, so little time. It's flat-out overwhelming out there in the world of nutrition. You've likely seen a dozen different diets splashed across your social media feed, all of them endorsed by "experts." There's carnivore, keto, Atkins, vegan, vegetarian, pescatarian, paleo, Mediterranean . . . it's nonstop. Diets are like opinions . . . everyone has one.

There's nothing inherently wrong with any of these ways of eating. They all have their pros and cons. The problem is when we try to make any one of them a universal prescription for everyone. I've never taken a hard stance on one particular way of eating because your body is not the same as your best friend's, your neighbor's, or that of the influencer you follow on social media. It all depends on your labs, and how you as an individual can tolerate carbohydrates and process and digest fats. You will need to do some experimenting to find out what works best for you, your thyroid, and your metabolism.

The Carnivore Diet

I'll start with the carnivore diet since it's probably the most extreme and most controversial on the spectrum. You eat only animal foods: meat, poultry, fish, eggs, and sometimes dairy products. No vegetables, no fruit, no grains . . . maybe some dark chocolate or honey here and there, but that's it. Many proponents of the carnivore diet swear by its inflammation-reducing capabilities, which is a big deal when you have Hashimoto's or other autoimmune conditions. By removing plants, you're also removing many potential gut irritants such as lectins, oxalates, and phytates. For people with severe gut permeability or histamine issues, this diet not only can simplify what they can eat and tolerate, but can also reduce or eliminate GI symptoms.

I've seen patients with raging autoimmunity problems, skin issues, and chronic bloating go on the carnivore diet for thirty to ninety days and finally feel normal again. Their body gets a break from constant immune triggers and can calm down enough to let them start healing.

But the carnivore diet isn't for everyone long term. You have to pay close attention to your micronutrients, including magnesium, vitamin C, and potassium. And you need to make sure you're eating from nose to tail if you want to cover all your nutrient bases. Yes, that means organ meats! Remember those liver and onions that your mom tried to bribe you into eating? She was actually onto something. Organ meats have higher concentrations of trace minerals, iron, zinc, selenium, B vitamins, and often vitamin A than muscle meat.[8]

Some carnivore diets will recommend reintroducing small amounts of carbohydrates in the form of fruits or root vegetables once your gut calms down. You don't have to go crazy and revert to salad and bread-sticks at Olive Garden; instead, try adding berries and see how you feel. Over time, you can find the right balance that works for you.

The Keto Diet

Although it has reached new heights of popularity in recent years, the keto diet has been around forever. It was first used in the 1920s as a ther-apeutic diet for epilepsy, but these days most people know it as a tool for weight loss, reversing insulin resistance, and calming inflammation. The keto diet is a low-carbohydrate, high-fat approach to eating that shifts your body's metabolism away from using carbs or glucose for energy to burning fat for fuel instead. In the world of cancer treatment, research suggests that a ketogenic diet can be used to create an unfavorable envi-ronment for cancer cells by depriving them of glucose.[9]

For good thyroid health, the keto diet can be incredibly helpful if you do it the right way. When you cut your consumption of carbs way down, your insulin level drops, your body switches to burning fat for fuel, and it starts producing ketones. Ketones are a by-product of breaking down fat for energy, and at low to moderate levels, they are anti-inflammatory and can help keep your blood sugar steady instead of spiking and crashing all day long. Lowering systemic, bodywide inflammation, as we know, takes pressure off both your thyroid and your adrenals.

There is some concern, however, that severely restricting carbs can impair T4 to T3 conversion.[10] A low-carb diet can reduce the activity of the deiodinase enzymes that convert T4 to T3, and lower insulin levels can also inhibit conversion. My feeling, however, is that if your thyroid is optimized and you've got T3 on board, any little dip you might see in conversion isn't a deal breaker. The biosynthetic T3 you are already tak-ing overrides any concerns.

There isn't just one way to do keto. My favorite is a higher-protein ver-sion. I don't like when people on the keto diet are scared of protein and eat only bacon and cheese. You need protein. Keeping carbs low while also eating plenty of lean, high-quality protein such as grass-fed beef, bison, venison, chicken, turkey, fish, and eggs or a high-quality beef isolate protein powder gives you the best of both worlds: You still make ketones, but you also have the amino acids needed to keep your muscle, repair your tissues, and support healthy thyroid conversion.

I'm also a fan of a cyclical keto approach, and I even created a mini-course called "Keto for the Week." The way it works is simple: Stay keto or low carb during the week, and then on one or two days over the weekend, increase your carb consumption a bit. This is not a "cheat day," or a loading up on gluten-free pizza and brownies day. It's adding a sweet potato or another nutrient-dense, complex carb to slightly bump up your complex carbs and fiber. That small bump in carbohydrates keeps your body guessing and your enzymes and insulin working and helps prevent your T3 from dipping over time.

Here's my advice: If you want to try the keto or carnivore diet, keep an eye on your labs. Watch your free T3, reverse T3, and cortisol. If you start feeling cold or tired or notice your hair shedding more than usual, it's a sign that you may be having T3 conversion problems. In that case, get your labs checked, and if your free T3 has dropped, adjust your dose or make sure you're converting properly. If your reverse T3 has climbed, check your cortisol and insulin levels, make medication adjustments, and try to address nutrient deficiencies. If a keto or carnivore diet is your thing, you should be able to keep your low-carb lifestyle as long as you adjust in other ways.

The Paleo Diet

The paleo diet is the one diet about which I don't really have any concerns, and for thyroid health, it is one of your best options. It's naturally gluten free, focuses on real food, and makes protein the star. It avoids grains, which are inflammatory, and it also takes out processed foods, legumes, dairy products, refined sugar, and seed oils. What you're left with is simple and powerful: meat, fish, eggs, vegetables, fruit, nuts, and healthy fats. The paleo diet can lean a little heavily on sugar with foods such as honey and dates, but it also puts a big emphasis on quality fats. The best part? The food tastes amazing. Paleo recipes are the kind of meals that even picky eaters eat without complaint.

For thyroid health, the paleo diet works beautifully. It lowers inflammation, supports your gut, and loads you up with nutrients. You naturally get more zinc, selenium, and iodine, three of the most important nutrients for thyroid function, just by following the plan.

If you're looking for something sustainable, the paleo diet is one of the easiest long-term approaches. It doesn't feel overly restrictive once you get used to it. It's just real food that leaves you feeling full, nourished, and energized.

The Mediterranean Diet

There's not much bad to say about the Mediterranean diet, either. It emphasizes plant-based foods such as fruits, vegetables, whole grains, legumes, and nuts, so it is full of healthy fats and antioxidants, and it also incorporates moderate amounts of fish, poultry, dairy products, and eggs, while being low in processed foods and sugar. It is also one of the best-studied diets, and research links it to better heart health, lower inflammation, and a host of other benefits across a variety of different health conditions.[11]

The only caution I'll add about the Mediterranean diet is to watch your carbohydrate intake, especially if you struggle with blood sugar swings. This diet includes bread, pasta, and grains, which can be too much if your insulin is already an issue. And if you have thyroid-related autoimmunity or osteoarthritis, you will need to skip the wheat and gluten-containing grains entirely, even if you follow other aspects of the Mediterranean plan.

Vegan and Vegetarian Diets

I'm going to be blunt: If you're eating this way for ethical or spiritual reasons, I respect that. But you still need to look at your lab work and be honest about whether your beliefs are serving your health.

Plant-based diets can be high in carbohydrates, even if you're eating whole foods. Many vegans rely on grains and legumes as their primary sources of protein, but in reality, these foods are mostly carbs. Furthermore, the amount of grains and legumes that you need to consume to achieve what I consider to be an adequate amount of protein is quite large. Over time, this can lead to all the same problems we see with any carb-heavy diet: blood sugar dysregulation, insulin resistance, and nutrient deficiencies. It won't surprise you that this also puts stress on your thyroid.

My patient Maya had been a lifelong vegan, deeply committed to her belief system and cultural roots. An Ayurveda practitioner who had dedicated her studies to understanding how food, herbs, and lifestyle can impact healing, she was disciplined, intentional, and absolutely dedicated to wellness. But when we ran her labs, the truth was undeniable: She was full-blown diabetic, and her blood sugar was out of control. Her thyroid was also underperforming. She was doing everything she could within her vegan framework to be healthy, but the way she was eating was pushing her body toward disease. I asked her to trust me.

We optimized her thyroid, but Maya also had to face the reality that her diet was not working for her body. This was not an easy shift for her, given her background, but she agreed to start incorporating animal-based proteins into her diet very slowly. And that was when things began to change. Almost immediately, her energy picked up, her mind felt clearer, and her blood sugar started to stabilize. Over time, her labs improved. Her thyroid responded better, and her blood sugar came down. She reported feeling lighter and more vibrant than she had in years.

This wasn't about abandoning her values or culture; it was about giving her body what it was missing so it could function the way it was meant to. And the transformation was the proof she needed. With that one small shift, adding back in the protein her body was starving for, she got her health, her strength, and her vitality back.

If you choose to eat vegan or vegetarian because it aligns with your beliefs, that's your decision. Just know that it takes a lot of extra effort to get enough protein, B$_{12}$, iron, zinc, selenium, iodine, and omega-3 fats, all of which are critical for thyroid health. You need to be willing to supplement aggressively and monitor your labs regularly.

You also need to ask yourself, "Is my belief system more important than my body?" and make your decision based on the answer.

The Paleto Diet: The Best of Both Worlds

If I had to pick the perfect way of eating for hypothyroid patients, it would be what I call the "paleto" diet: paleo plus keto. And no, it's not an official diet (yet), but it should be. When you look at the paleo diet, the concept is: gluten free, no grains, and no dairy products, with a focus on high-quality grass-fed proteins, healthy fats, and clean carbohydrates such as root vegetables and sweet potatoes. It's nutrient dense, but for people with insulin resistance, the levels of carbs and sugars can be too high.

Then there is the keto diet: low carb, high fat, lots of protein. But here's the problem. Too many people do "dirty keto." They start every morning with heavy whipping cream in their coffee, make casseroles with five types of cheese, eat bacon all day, and end the night with high-fat coconut milk pudding. I've done that myself. I've started the day with heavy cream, kept piling on the cheese, eaten ample amounts of bacon with a smile on my face, and wondered why I was gaining weight. The truth is, fat has more calories than any other macronutrient. Even if you eat low carb, if you're taking in 3,000 calories a day but burning only 2,000, the math says you are going to gain weight.

Here's where the paleto diet comes in. When you blend the high-quality food focus of the paleo diet with the low-carb, moderate-fat approach of the keto diet, you hit the sweet spot. Many people need some keto principles woven into their paleo in order to feel their best, including the option for high-quality dairy. With paleto, you get the anti-inflammatory benefits of the keto diet without drowning in poor-quality fats. You get the nutrient density of the paleo diet without overdoing carbs. What does that give you? Steady energy, balanced blood sugar, less inflammation, and better support for thyroid conversion.

• • •

Whatever diet you choose, remember that there is no magic diet that will cure your thyroid. There is no one-size-fits-all solution. You still need enough protein to maintain muscle and repair tissues, enough healthy fats to support your hormones, and enough nutrient density to heal. This isn't about subscribing to a label or living in a box; it's about building an eating style that helps you feel clear, energized, and strong. If you keep that as your North Star, you'll find the approach that works best for you.

Chapter 12

Lift Heavy Sh*t

A t our clinic, we have a saying: "You have to lift heavy sh*t." I'm not suggesting you need to throw your back out or blow out a knee trying to squat three hundred pounds, but exercise—the *right* kind of exercise—has a part to play in maintaining your thyroid health as you go forward.

Believe it or not, thanks to our gym-obsessed culture, a lot of women today are overexercising. I'm talking to you, Cardio Queens. I see you on your Peloton grinding through an hour of cardio, and I get it. I used to be that person, too. As I told you, my obsession with fitness started at the ripe old age of twelve, in my living room with Jane Fonda aerobics tapes. By age fifteen, I had joined my first gym, and of course I went straight to step classes and the StairMaster. I wouldn't leave until I'd done at least an hour.

Before long I was certified to teach step, and cardio was always daily and mandatory. Somewhere along the way, someone—maybe it was Jane Fonda or even Richard Simmons—convinced me that cardio was the holy grail. Sure, if I had extra time, I'd wander over to the Nautilus machines or pick up a few weights, but cardio was always the priority.

I'm not knocking the benefits of cardiovascular exercise entirely. But the high heart rates that come with cardio put stress on the body in ways that are often overlooked. That's because when your heart rate goes up, your cortisol level goes up, too. Essentially, your body's fight-or-flight response kicks in to power you through a physically demanding burst of activity. And an elevated cortisol level, as we know, can drive up reverse T3 and create a less-than-ideal environment for thyroid function.

Too much cardio not only pumps cortisol into your body, it can also sabotage your attempts at building muscle. When your heart rate goes up and remains there for an extended period of time, as during high-intensity cardio workouts such as spinning or CrossFit, your body is forced to shift to an alternate metabolism to fuel your activity. You stop burning fat (a slower process) and instead burn glucose, which is more quickly converted to ATP. If your blood sugar is low or you start your workout in a fasted state, your body is forced to pull glucose from backup stores inside your muscles. And when those stores are depleted, your body doesn't switch back to burning fat—instead, it starts breaking down proteins in the muscles.

When I was prepping for shows during my competition days, the trainers I worked with had me doing two cardio sessions a day on top of all my weight training. I'd spend hours in the gym lifting to build strong, lean muscle, only to tear it down with cardio right after. The constant physical stress on my body didn't make me leaner; in fact, it layered more fat onto my frame. When I think about it now, it sounds crazy, but at the time I truly believed that was the way to stay fit and healthy.

About six years ago, I quit doing cardio altogether. And when I say quit, I mean completely. The only "cardio" I do now is five to ten minutes of all-out sprints on an Airdyne bike or a few rounds of hammering a heavy bag. My workouts now are built around lifting heavy shit and doing resistance training with intention. Honestly, nothing gets your heart rate up like picking up a loaded barbell from the ground. It's way more effective than any treadmill or stair climber, while keeping cortisol and systemic inflammation down.

Now, at fifty-one, I have the physique I used to dream about: the capped shoulders I always wanted, visible biceps. I have deep cuts in my quads and a rounder butt than I had in my twenties, when I was literally running my ass off. I have more muscle now than I did when I was power lifting, and my body composition is better than ever. More muscle means a better metabolism and better insulin sensitivity, which supports my thyroid. And I made it all happen without doing cardio.

I'm not telling you to avoid doing exercise that gets your heart rate up; I'm just telling you that you don't need hours of steady-state cardio to make it happen. You can push your heart rate plenty just by lifting weights, but the built-in rest time between sets in resistance training allows your heart rate to settle and keeps your cortisol levels down. You can toss in a few burpees between sets or hit ten short sprints on a bike and get more out of those minutes than you ever will by slogging away on a treadmill. And here's the truth: If your heart rate isn't rising when you strength train, either you're not challenging yourself enough in terms of weight load, or you're spending too much time chatting with your gym buddies between sets.

Too many people accept muscle loss as a part of aging, but when you lift heavy shit consistently, you can slow that loss down or even reverse it and make gains. Building and holding on to muscle not only gives you a better metabolism, which helps your thyroid, it also protects your bones, lowers your risk of heart disease and stroke, helps you live longer, and makes a huge difference in your quality of life.[1] In fact, as I mentioned previously, some people say that muscle is your organ of longevity. It's what keeps you strong, stable, and able to do the things you love. If you don't maintain it, you put your health and independence on the line.

The Power of Strength Training

Studies show that strength training or resistance training is the best way to build and maintain muscle.[2] So pick up some weights, use machines, use TRX or resistance bands, or use your own body weight, but give your muscles some kind of resistance. If you really want to age well and live independently until the day you die, and if you want to optimize your metabolism so that your thyroid functions beautifully forever more, resistance training needs to be a regular part of your life.

Here are some additional ways in which strength training supports your body.

Increased Bone Density and Osteoporosis Prevention

Weight-bearing exercise, such as lifting heavy weights, increases bone density.[3] When you put load and tension on your bones by lifting weights or doing resistance exercise, that stress on the bone sends a signal to your osteoblasts, the bone-building cells, to lay down new bone tissue. Over time, this increases your bone mineral density and makes your bones stronger and more resistant to fractures. This is why strength training is one of the most effective ways to prevent osteoporosis. It literally tells your body, "Hey, we need stronger bones to handle this load," and your body responds by building them.

Protection of Your Internal Organs

Building muscle is not just about looking toned in your jeans. Muscle is your suit of armor. Hello, modern-day Joan of Arc! When you build muscle, you are putting added protection around your body. Strong muscles wrap around your torso and spine like a shield, giving you a cushion that absorbs impact if you fall or get knocked around. Your core and back muscles stabilize your spine and protect the delicate structures inside your abdominal cavity. Muscle is a built-in shock absorber, keeping your organs and bones safe throughout the activities of daily life.

Power and Strength

When you have muscle, you don't just look stronger—you are stronger. You can carry heavy grocery bags, hoist your suitcase up into the overhead bin on an airplane, or pick up your kid or grandkid without a second thought. More than that, muscle gives you confidence. It makes you that badass woman who knows she can kick someone's ass if she ever has to. I'm not suggesting that you get bulky. I just want you to reclaim your strength, protection, and independence. Building muscle is saying, "I am not fragile, and I am not going quietly into old age."

Good Heart Health and Circulation

Lifting heavy shit is one of the best things you can do for your heart. When you lift, your muscles contract and relax, and that action boosts your circulation and pumps blood back to your heart more efficiently. It keeps your arteries flexible and lowers the resistance in your blood vessels. Over time, consistent strength training can bring your blood pressure down and improve your overall heart health.[4] It also increases stroke volume—a fancy way of saying your heart pumps more blood with each beat. The result is a stronger, more efficient heart that doesn't have to work as hard to keep you going.

Lower Insulin Sensitivity and Diabetes Prevention

Lift heavy sh*t training also changes the way your body handles blood sugar. Bigger, stronger, sexier muscles store more glucose as glycogen, which means they pull glucose out of your bloodstream and keep your blood sugar level steady. Think of your muscles as being like a sponge: The more muscle you have, the more glucose (sugar) they soak up. That keeps your insulin stable, lowers your blood sugar, and protects you from insulin resistance—which, as we know, impacts thyroid health—and type 2 diabetes.

Protein Reservoir and Recovery

Muscle is also like a storage bank for amino acids. When your body needs extra protein to heal a wound, fight off an infection, or recover from surgery, it taps into that bank. The more muscle you have, the bigger your reserve of these critical building blocks. That's why people with more muscle bounce back faster, heal quicker, and come out stronger when life knocks them down.

This is why it's so important to include sufficient protein in your diet.

The protein you consume supplies the raw material, and lifting tells your body to put that material to use. Together they create the kind of muscle that not only keeps you strong from day to day but also gives your body the reserves it needs when life throws challenges your way.

Increased Metabolic Rate and Calorie Burning

If everything else I've said about muscle hasn't grabbed your attention, this will: More muscle means better metabolism and a higher basal metabolic rate.[5] Put simply, more muscle means you burn more calories and more fat, way more than you would without it.

Muscle is metabolically active in a way fat never will be. Every pound of muscle burns energy just to exist. That means that the more muscle you carry, the more fat you burn at rest while you're sitting at your desk, driving in your car, or even watching Netflix at night.

This is why lifting heavy shit matters so much for fat loss and keeping it off. You're not just burning calories during the workout, you're creating a body that keeps burning calories for you all day long. Muscle gives you the edge. It makes you a fat-burning machine instead of a fat-storing one, so you don't have to torture yourself with endless dietary restrictions or feel miserable on another diet.

Here's the best part. When you build muscle, you have more wiggle room. You can enjoy the sweet potato fries or the gluten-free pizza on the weekend without freaking out about being five pounds heavier on Monday. That's the gift muscle gives you.

Improved Mood and Greater Confidence

Any kind of physical activity, but especially strength training, can boost your mood. Let's face it, you feel like a badass when you have a great workout. When you lift five pounds more than you did last week, when you get one more rep in that biceps curl, when you do one more push-up than you've ever done before, it kicks off your day. It makes you feel powerful.

Getting Started

Here's the thing: You can build muscle at any age. It takes an optimized thyroid, the right balance of hormones, and proper nutrition that includes enough protein and amino acids to support muscle growth. But the most important part is that you start lifting heavy shit, no matter how old you are.

What you perceive as heavy is relative. It depends on your body, any injuries you may have, and your current strength level. If you are new to exercise, start slowly with light weights or simple resistance work. Even a few sessions with a personal trainer can help you learn safe form and set up a routine you can stick with, whether at a gym or at home. If a trainer is not an option, there are plenty of great free resources. My friend and trainer Lisa Maximus created an incredible app called Maximus Strong that truly has everything you need. You can pick the perfect workout that meets you where you are, then take it to the gym and follow along with weights and machines, roll with your garage setup, or do it at home with zero equipment. It makes strength training simple, adaptable, and easy to follow at any fitness level. Think of it as having a trainer in your pocket.

The important thing is not just to build strength; you also need to develop power. Muscle power—that is, how fast and efficiently you can move—is often even more important for daily living and functional independence than raw strength is. Quicker movements against resistance, such as air squats with your own body weight or jump squats if your joints are healthy, develop that power. These fast-twitch movements train your nervous system to recruit muscle fibers quickly, which is critical for preventing falls and staying capable as you get older.

You can work on developing power anywhere. When you are climbing stairs, push off the step as quickly as possible while holding the handrail for safety. Mix these kinds of movements into your routine along with your heavy lifting, and you are not just exercising, you are building resilience. You are protecting your bones, your heart, your metabolism, your thyroid, and your future.

The real key to building muscle at any age is consistency. As we get older, we lose strength and size faster if we take long breaks from training. Staying consistent with both movement and resistance work is how you will keep the muscle you build and continue to progress.

So get off the hamster wheel. Pick up something heavy. Feel your heart rate climb. Feel your muscles work. And remember, you are never too old, too out of shape, or too far gone to start. Now that we've fixed your thyroid and you are getting your life back, this is how you reclaim your strength. This is how you feel like a badass again.

Chapter 13

Lower Your Toxic Load: Simple Steps to Detox Naturally

———

I'll never forget the time I walked into an Airbnb after a long day of travel. The door swung open, and it was like getting punched in the face by the most pungent, flowery smell I'd ever encountered. I'm talking about an invisible wall of fragrance that hit me right between the eyes.

I looked around and realized why. There weren't just one or two plug-in air fresheners in that house—there were no fewer than ten. Every room had a glowing little chemical bomb pumping synthetic fragrance into the air.

I unplugged every one of them and stuck them in a closet. But even then, the smell lingered for the next twenty-four hours, clinging to my clothes and hair, and to the sheets. What came next was the waves of a pounding headache, water retention, and thick brain fog. My body just didn't want to work. Even though the effect was temporary, I could feel that the exposure to the chemicals was punching my thyroid in the face. Or rather, punching every cell in my body in the face.

What's wild is that most people wouldn't think twice about it. We've been trained to believe that everything needs to smell better than it does. We think we need some kind of artificial fragrance flowing over the reality of our lives. It's obvious from the air freshener plug-ins in every hallway to the sweet pea and salted caramel body sprays you douse yourself with after a shower. From the vanilla bean lotion that is

supposed to calm your nerves to the lavender linen spray that supposedly helps you sleep.

I'm going to say what no one else will: All those pretty smells are a
cocktail of chemicals. They're not benign. They're not harmless. They're
endocrine disruptors that are inhaled, absorbed through your skin, and
stored in your tissues.[1] They layer up over time until you're sitting there
wondering why your thyroid isn't working, you feel puffy and inflamed,
and your brain feels as though it's packed in wet cotton.

You can be doing everything right—dialing in your thyroid meds,
cleaning up your diet, choosing strength training instead of spin class—
and still feel like you're wading through mud every day. If that's you, it's
time to look at the hidden factor nobody wants to talk about: the toxins
silently trashing your thyroid.

We live in a world our grandparents couldn't have imagined. There
are over eighty thousand chemicals approved for use in the United States
alone. They're in our food, water, air, cleaning supplies, personal care
products, receipts, furniture, cookware, and clothing. We are swimming
in a chemical soup, and as I talked about in chapter 3, your thyroid is one
of the first casualties.

The small, butterfly-shaped gland sitting at the base of your neck is
like a canary in the coal mine. It picks up signals from your environment, and when the load gets too heavy, it slows everything down in
an attempt to protect you. However, if you're serious about protecting
your thyroid, you should try to avoid the following toxins whenever
you can.

1. **The toxic halogens: fluorine, chlorine, and bromine.** These chemicals
   are structurally similar to iodine, and when you're exposed to them
   in high amounts, as with fluoride in your tap water or toothpaste or
   bromine in baked goods and soft drinks, they can displace iodine
   in your thyroid tissue.[2] Imagine trying to build a house with rotten
   wood. That's what your thyroid is doing when it tries to produce T4
   and T3 using one of these other halogens instead of iodine. Over

time, this can lead to iodine deficiency in the gland, reducing its hormone output and triggering hypothyroidism.

Here are some steps you can take to avoid these toxins: Choose a high-quality water filter that removes fluoride and chlorine, avoid drinking unfiltered tap water, skip fluoride toothpaste, avoid brominated vegetable oils in soft drinks, choose organic bread products (or make your own) that do not use brominated dough conditioners, don't sit in chlorinated hot tubs, and rinse off right after swimming in a chlorinated pool. And . . . take extra iodine if you *are* exposed.

2. **Heavy metals, such as mercury, lead, arsenic, and cadmium.** These are some of the toxins most disruptive to your thyroid. They interfere with hormone production, hormone conversion, and the communication between your thyroid and your brain.[3] The frustrating part is that you come into contact with them far more often than you may think.

   Mercury in particular has a high affinity for the enzymes your body needs to convert T4 to T3. When mercury binds up those enzymes, your conversion slows to a crawl,[4] and suddenly you have plenty of T4 but not enough of the active T3 that fuels your metabolism, mood, and energy. Lead damages the thyroid follicular cells,[5] the ones that produce thyroid hormones. Arsenic interferes with thyroid hormone metabolism and has been linked to changes in TSH and T4 levels.[6] Cadmium disrupts the entire hypothalamic-pituitary-thyroid (HPT) axis,[7] which throws off the feedback loops your hormones rely on for balance.

   Where do these heavy metals come from, and how can we avoid them?

   Mercury, as you may already know, is present in large fish such as tuna, swordfish, king mackerel, and tilefish because they naturally accumulate more mercury, being higher on the food chain. It is also found in dental amalgam fillings, which release small amounts of mercury vapor whenever you chew or grind your teeth. Some imported cosmetics, especially skin-lightening products, contain mercury as a preservative. Mercury can also be present in air pollution from coal burning and then settle into water and soil.

To avoid mercury, choose low-mercury fish such as salmon, sardines, trout, and cod. If you have old amalgam fillings, have them removed only by a qualified biologic dentist to prevent exposure during removal. Avoid questionable imported cosmetics, and use a high-quality water filter if you live in or near an industrial region.

Lead is found in older homes built before 1978, in lead-based paint that flakes off and turns into dust as it ages. Older plumbing systems can leach lead into drinking water, especially when hot water runs through pipes that contain lead solder. Some inexpensive ceramic dishes and mugs, especially those with bright glazes, may contain lead that leaches into food. Lead can also be present in soil near highways, old buildings, and industrial sites, as well as in some imported spices. There have also been a number of food recalls in recent years, where lead has been found in alarming concentrations in products such as spices, chocolate, and baby formula.

To avoid lead, use a water filter that is certified to remove lead, avoid chipped or low-quality ceramic dishes, let cold water run before drinking if you live in an older home, wash your hands often during remodeling projects, and choose well-tested spices from reputable manufacturers.

Arsenic is naturally present in soil and water, but certain crops absorb more of it than others. Rice is a major dietary source because it grows in standing water, which traps arsenic. Apple juice and grape juice often contain measurable levels as well. Some areas of the country have arsenic in the groundwater, and older pressure-treated wood can contain arsenic-based chemicals.

To avoid arsenic, choose rice from California or basmati rice from India, which tend to have lower arsenic content. Rinse rice thoroughly, and cook it in extra water that you then drain off. Filter your water if you live in a region with known arsenic issues. Limit your consumption of fruit juices, or choose brands that publicly share their heavy metal testing results. Avoid using old pressure-treated lumber in garden beds where you grow food.

Cadmium occurs in cigarette smoke, contaminated soil, non-organic leafy greens, shellfish, and some cocoa powders. It also appears in certain cheap metal jewelry or cookware. Cadmium accumulates in soil due to industrial pollution and phosphate fertilizers, which means that plants grown in these soils can absorb it.

To avoid cadmium, avoid smoking and secondhand smoke entirely, choose organic leafy greens when possible, buy cocoa products from companies that test for heavy metals, avoid cheap metal cookware and jewelry with unknown sourcing, and rinse all your produce well to remove soil residue.

Heavy metals are everywhere, but you do not need to fear them. You just need to know where they hide so you can reduce your exposure and take pressure off your thyroid, your detox pathways, and your entire hormonal system.

3. **Plastics: BPA (bisphenol A), BPS (bisphenol S), and phthalates.** Bisphenol A (BPA) and its cousin bisphenol S (BPS) are synthetic chemicals used in plastics and thermal paper, and they are powerful endocrine disruptors that have a direct impact on thyroid function.[8] BPA has long been used in food and beverage packaging, water bottles, can linings, and especially paper receipts. As BPA came under public scrutiny, many companies simply replaced it with BPS, a nearly identical compound that is just as hormonally disruptive.

Both BPA and BPS interfere with thyroid hormone activity on multiple levels: They block thyroid hormone receptors so T3 cannot do its job inside your cells, impair the conversion of T4 to T3, increase reverse T3, and disrupt signaling along the hypothalamic-pituitary-thyroid (HPT) axis.[9] They can also contribute to autoimmune activation in those who are predisposed to Hashimoto's, making them particularly problematic for anyone already dealing with thyroid dysfunction.

Exposure is widespread because BPA and BPS are found in thermal paper receipts from grocery stores, gas stations, pharmacies, restaurants, and ATMs. Simply holding a receipt for a few seconds transfers these chemicals to the skin, and as luck would have it, using hand sanitizer beforehand increases absorption dramatically. They also appear in plastics such as water bottles, storage containers, utensils, food packaging, and shaker bottles, as well as in many canned foods due to the lining inside the can. Because receipts are recycled with other paper products, even household items such as toilet paper, paper towels, and napkins can contain trace amounts. Some personal care and household products also use BPA- or BPS-containing plastic components, adding to everyday exposure.

Minimizing contact does not require perfection, just strategy. Avoid handling receipts whenever possible, and ask for digital versions instead. Never touch receipts after using hand sanitizer or lotion. Use glass or stainless-steel water bottles, choose BPA- and BPS-free storage containers, and avoid heating food in plastic. Reduce your canned food intake or choose brands labeled as BPA free, although many still use BPS. Opt for fresh or frozen foods when you can. Small, consistent steps add up and can significantly reduce your endocrine-disrupting load, which is crucial when you are trying to optimize thyroid function, lower inflammation, and regain metabolic balance.

4. **Pesticides and herbicides.** Pesticides and herbicides deliver another huge hit to your thyroid, and most people have no clue how often they're being exposed. These chemicals are everywhere: They are sprayed on our food, our lawns, our parks, and the soccer fields our kids play on, and they drift right into the air you breathe. They don't politely stay on the outside of a strawberry; they sink into the fruit,

make their way into your body, and start messing with your thyroid hormone production.

Organophosphate pesticides are the worst offenders. They block thyroid peroxidase,[10] the enzyme that starts the hormone production process. This is the moment your thyroid takes iodine and attaches it to tyrosine. If that step is interrupted, the assembly line slows down, and you won't be making enough hormone.

Other pesticides cause trouble in different ways. Some compete with iodine, so your thyroid has to fight for the raw materials it needs.[11] Some disrupt the communication between your brain and your thyroid, so your body cannot get an accurate read on what needs to be produced.[12] And a lot of these chemicals irritate your gut lining or throw off your gut bacteria.[13] Since a good chunk of T4 to T3 conversion happens in the gut, that disruption means you can be walking around with low T3 even if you are technically producing enough T4. No wonder you feel awful.

And here's the part no one wants to hear: You are being exposed even if you eat organic and try to live clean. These chemicals are on golf courses, playgrounds, parks, school grounds, and every pristine landscaped lawn your dog walks past. They drift in the air, they end up in household dust, and they absolutely show up in water supplies. You can be doing everything right and still end up being exposed.

You don't have to move to the mountains and grow your own food, but you can absolutely reduce your toxic load. Buy organic whenever you can, especially the highest-residue foods. The Dirty Dozen is a list published by the Environmental Working Group of the twelve conventionally grown fruits and vegetables with the highest pesticide residues: spinach, strawberries, dark leafy greens (kale, collard, and mustard), grapes, peaches, cherries, nectarines, pears, apples, blackberries, blueberries, and potatoes. Buy these organic whenever possible and wash any produce you purchase like you mean it. Filter your water with a filter that actually works. Stop using weed killers on your lawn. And when you see those little signs at a park saying the ground was just treated, do not let your kids or your dog run all over it. Give it time.

Adopting all these small habits will lighten the load on your thyroid. When your body is not swimming in chemicals that block hormone production and conversion, your body will start working the way it should. You will feel clearer, lighter, calmer, and more like yourself again. This is one of those areas in which little changes truly add up.

5. **Synthetic fragrances.** We need to be more aware of synthetic fragrances: the plug-ins, candles, sprays, dryer sheets, scented laundry detergents, and air fresheners that are in nearly every home and public space. These products contain phthalates and volatile organic compounds (VOCs) that you inhale and absorb through your skin. Phthalates in synthetic fragrances can bind to thyroid hormone receptors, disrupting normal signaling.[14] VOCs trigger inflammation and oxidative stress,[15] which damage thyroid cells over time. For some people, even short-term exposure can cause headaches, swelling of mucous membranes or the respiratory tract, fatigue, and brain fog, just as it did to me in that Airbnb. For others, it's a constant low-grade assault that slowly chips away at their energy, mood, and metabolism.

   You'd be shocked by how many chemicals you absorb through your skin and lungs. Investing in an air scrubber such as a Jaspr can significantly reduce your exposure to these airborne endocrine disruptors. More on this below.

6. **Flame retardants (polybrominated diphenyl ethers, or PBDEs).** These are chemicals found in things such as mattresses, upholstered furniture, and electronics. Over time, they build up in your fat tissue and slowly leak out into the rest of your body. They can attach to thyroxine-binding globulin (TBG) and other proteins that carry thyroid hormones throughout your body, which lowers your amount of free T4 and keeps your thyroid receptors from working properly.[16]

Studies have shown that higher blood levels of PBDEs are linked to more cases of hypothyroidism, especially in women.[17] These include a 2016 study in the *Journal of Clinical Endocrinology and Metabolism* and a 2016 study in *Environmental Health*, both of which confirmed a positive association between PBDEs in blood serum and thyroid disease in women, especially in postmenopausal women.

. . .

It's easy to feel overwhelmed when you realize how many ways toxins sneak into your body. But I'm not writing this to scare you into panic mode or make you think you have to move to a cabin in the woods and live off rainwater. Remember the 80/20 rule. This is about awareness and making better choices when you can.

Your liver and detox pathways are your body's built-in cleaning crew (think of detox pathways as your body's interstate highways used to eliminate waste and toxins). But if you're under chronic stress, eating processed food, and running on caffeine, your detox systems will be operating at half capacity. That toxic burden starts to build up, and eventually it spills over into your thyroid. There are ways you can combat your exposures, but this is not about a quick fix. I cringe when I see people doing another trendy detox tea or a weeklong juice cleanse. You don't need a starvation protocol; you need to lower your exposure, support your detox highway, and let your body do what it's meant to do.

That starts with your daily choices. Filter your water. Get rid of your nonstick pans. Stop microwaving plastic containers. Buy organic when you can, especially the Dirty Dozen. Switch out your toxic cleaning and skin care products. Swap out air fresheners and scented candles for essential oils or an air purifier.

Support your liver with real food. Get enough protein so your body has the amino acids it needs to fuel the detoxification process. Make sure you're pooping every day. You can't detox if you're constipated; those toxins will just be reabsorbed and recirculate, wreaking more havoc on your thyroid.

Sweating matters, too. Your skin is your paramount organ of elimination. Sauna, exercise, and even a hot bath with Epsom salts can help pull toxins out of your tissues and move them out of your body. I'll talk more about these in chapter 15.

Remember, you don't have to be perfect about detoxing for it to have an impact. This isn't about never touching a paper receipt again or living in fear that you'll have to. It's about reducing your cumulative load over time. Every little shift you make lowers the burden on your thyroid.

Your thyroid doesn't need a fad Beyoncé cayenne pepper and lemon cleanse. It needs you to stop flooding it with chemicals and give your detox pathways the support they need. You can't control every toxin in your environment, but you can control a lot more than you think and you can significantly lower your toxic burden. And when you lower that burden, you will give your thyroid the breathing room to function the way it was designed to. That's how you move from surviving to thriving.

Your Detox Baseline: Clean Air and Water

This combo might not sound sexy, but it's foundational. Air purifiers with HEPA filters help reduce VOCs, mold spores, and other airborne toxins that inflame your thyroid. I have three Jaspr air scrubbers in my home, and it's amazing how often they "kick on" when they detect particles of toxins in the air. It only reinforces how much we're exposed to on a daily basis: Using hair spray, cooking protein pancakes, or even having the windows open on a nice spring day will make my Jasprs get to work.

Similarly, a good water filter is one of the simplest but most powerful upgrades you can make for your thyroid. Your tap water carries chlorine, fluoride, and often traces of heavy metals. As you know by now, all three interfere with iodine uptake and hormone production. If your thyroid cannot pull in iodine, it cannot make hormones. It's that simple. And you would be shocked at how many people are struggling because of what is coming out of their faucet every single day.

The gold standard is a whole-house reverse osmosis (RO)

system. This gives you clean water at every tap, every shower, and every sink, and it removes the chemicals that disrupt not just your thyroid but your skin, your gut, and your overall detox pathways. When you shower in chlorinated or fluoridated water, you absorb those chemicals through your skin. You also inhale them in steam. A whole-house RO system takes that burden off your body whether you are drinking, cooking, or bathing.

If a whole-house RO system is not in the budget right now, I recommend at least getting a high-quality, under-sink filtration system for your drinking water. The cheap filters on the shelf at the grocery store are not enough. They make your water taste better, but they do not actually remove the endocrine disruptors that are blocking your thyroid from doing its job.

Clean water is foundational. It supports iodine uptake, hormone production, and even your gut since water quality affects your microbiome, too. It is one of those things you do once and then your entire body thanks you every day. If you do nothing else, start here.

Chapter 14

Flip Stress on Its Head: Your Thyroid's Guide to Not Giving a F*ck

You can eat the cleanest diet in the world, strength train with the best personal trainer, take the right supplements, and follow every other health guideline you come across. But if stress becomes a constant background presence in your life, your thyroid *will* pay the price.

We can't talk about stress without talking about the adrenal glands. Your adrenal glands sit on top of your kidneys and function as little stress sentinels, responsible for producing adrenaline and cortisol, two hormones designed to keep you alive when your body perceives a threat. Cortisol is the main player here, and while it is often demonized, it's not inherently bad. You need cortisol to wake up in the morning, manage inflammation (it has anti-inflammatory properties), and keep your blood sugar stable between meals.

But your cortisol level is meant to rise and fall, not stay stuck on high for long stretches of time. If your body is constantly in "threat" mode and stress becomes your everyday state, your cortisol level will remain high, keeping your body constantly amped up and primed for fight or flight. When you're rushing through your day, glued to your phone, and worrying about your finances while juggling your job, kids, and aging parents, your brain can't tell the difference between a looming work deadline and being chased by a tiger. The result is the same: a flood of cortisol.

High and steady cortisol output sets off a cascade of dysfunction all over your body. In the beginning, you feel wired but tired. You're exhausted but can't fall asleep. You wake up between 2:00 and 4:00 a.m. with your mind racing. Inflammation skyrockets, blood sugar becomes unstable. Your cravings shift; all of a sudden you want salt, carbs, sugar—anything that provides quick energy. You feel frazzled, exhausted, burned out. And no matter how clean you eat, your midsection holds on to fat because your body perceives a need to conserve resources.

That's the cortisol cascade in action: inflammation, blood sugar spikes and crashes, fat storage, poor-quality sleep. And once this pattern takes hold, it rarely stays in its own lane. It drags your thyroid into the mess, too.

The Adrenal-Thyroid Hormone Loop

Cortisol influences your thyroid in several ways. First, it reduces your pituitary gland's production of TSH, the signal that tells your thyroid to produce T4 and T3. Second, it also suppresses the activity of D1 and D2, the enzymes that convert T4 to T3. Even worse, excess cortisol can increase the production of reverse T3, the bouncer at the club that prevents active T3 from entering your cells, so that only adds to the mix.[1]

Additionally, stress can influence how your cells respond to the thyroid hormone you do have. When cortisol stays chronically elevated, your cells may actually reduce the number of thyroid receptors on their surface,[2] which means they can't receive the T3 that activates metabolism, energy, and other cellular functions. Combined, these changes can leave you feeling exhausted, heavy, and foggy, even if your lab results are "normal." But these symptoms are real, and they reflect a body trying to adapt to prolonged stress.

Think of your thyroid and adrenal systems as two sides of the same coin. When one shifts, the other adjusts to compensate. Chronic stress and overly active adrenals can nudge your thyroid toward sluggishness. Similarly, a slow thyroid can cause the adrenals to work harder, pumping out more cortisol and adrenaline just to keep you going. And around it goes.

Given this strong connection, it's easy to see why people assume that their adrenals are responsible for how they feel. The thinking is "If I can just fix my adrenals, everything else will fall into place." But that's often a misconception. There is a belief, even among some practitioners, that if you "fix the adrenals," your thyroid will magically heal itself, as if sprinkling some adrenal fairy dust onto your body will suddenly make your struggling thyroid pump out more T3.

Supporting your adrenals matters, but it's not the whole story. Stress management, good-quality sleep, and adrenal support can make a difference in how you feel, but if your thyroid has gone off track, they won't replace proper thyroid treatment. That's why the goal of this chapter is to help you get your stress under control so you can see how it impacts both your adrenals and your thyroid, not to convince you that an "adrenal reset" is the answer. Don't fall for the social media marketing tactics of influencers trying to sell you adrenal protocols as a one-step solution. In fact, more often than not, the opposite is true: When you optimize your thyroid, your adrenals often settle back into balance naturally—*if* you are not running yourself into the ground with constant stress, lack of sleep, overwork, and punishing exercise. You have to address your thyroid and your stress at the same time, because you can't outsupplement or outmedicate a life that is overloading your nervous system.

Testing Your Cortisol

The best way to check your adrenal health and cortisol production is through a four-point saliva cortisol panel rather than a blood test, which reflects only one moment in time. Cortisol's proper pattern is to be high in the morning, when its level naturally rises to wake you up. Then it gradually declines throughout the day and is low at night. That's what relaxes you and gets you ready to sleep. You can't sleep well if your cortisol level is high at night; that's when you get that wired but tired second wind that has you cleaning your house at 10:00 p.m. That's most likely due to elevated cortisol. Ideally, you test your saliva for cortisol at four different times throughout the day, look at the results, and address any highs or lows you see. If your cortisol is flatlined low or high, you will need to work with a knowledgeable practitioner because you *may* need medication to address the problem, but true adrenal burnout is rare. Nine times out of ten, you can reset your cortisol pattern through optimizing your thyroid and hormones and by implementing the stress-balancing strategies below.

Strategies for Reducing Stress

None of us should blame ourselves for being stressed, but if you feel as though your thyroid has betrayed you, it helps to consider what your body has been managing. Our modern lives are perfectly designed to keep us in constant fight-or-flight mode. No one leaves their work at the office when they go home at night anymore. We bring it home with us. And then there's the news, politics, celebrity drama, social media drama . . . It's harder than ever to escape the news or distance ourselves from people we'd prefer to avoid. Look at the relentless pressure you've been under: the sleepless nights, the constant hustle of multitasking, maybe dealing with unresolved anger or grief. So give yourself some grace. There is nothing inherently wrong with you. Your body is doing exactly what it was designed to do, trying to protect you in the only way it knows how.

The last thing I want to do is to make you feel stressed about stress affecting your thyroid! But awareness is powerful. Your body isn't fragile, it's a resilient, adaptable machine that works incredibly hard to keep you going. But as we've talked about throughout this book, if you ignore the signals long enough, your body will turn up the volume until you finally listen. So let's make a deal right here: We're all going to do what we can to ease our stress levels, create better habits, and give our bodies the breathing room they need to be healthy. But we're not going to stress about stress. That's not the goal. The goal is to work with your body, not fight against it.

Once you understand how stress hijacks your thyroid, you can start to make different choices. Sometimes it's as simple as creating better sleep hygiene or setting stronger boundaries around your time. Sometimes it's about learning to say no. Sometimes it means asking for help or letting go of the idea that you have to be everything to everyone. And sometimes it means you need to call in targeted support from supplements and practices that can help shift your body's response to stress.

Supplements for Stress

Adaptogenic herbs such as **ashwagandha**, which I talked about in chapter 9, and **rhodiola** can buffer the stress response. Both are available as supplements and can be taken in conjunction with thyroid medication. They can help support the adrenals and thus help the thyroid to function better.[3]

Phosphatidylserine is a human phospholipid that plays an essential role in brain function and may help regulate the body's response to stress by blunting the release of cortisol.[4] It can also be derived from certain plants and, as a supplement, can help lower nighttime cortisol and assist with falling asleep.[5]

Holy basil, also called tulsi, is one of my favorite calming adaptogens because it works gently and steadily. It helps regulate cortisol without sedating you, and it has a grounding effect on the nervous system.[6] Women who feel "on edge" or overstimulated often respond well to holy basil. It supports the body's ability to return to baseline after stress and can help quiet the internal chatter that refuses to settle.

Schisandra is another powerful adaptogen that supports the stress response while also helping your liver detox more efficiently. Because it supports both stress resilience and metabolic pathways,[7] it's especially helpful when stress has left you feeling fatigued, foggy, or inflamed. Many women describe schisandra as giving them a clearer, steadier energy without jitters or crashes.

Cordyceps is technically a mushroom, but it behaves like an adaptogen. It supports cellular energy, endurance, and adrenal resilience.[8] When you've pushed yourself too hard for too long and feel depleted, cordyceps helps your body recover its ability to produce steady energy again. It's especially supportive if stress has drained your stamina or you feel physically drained by daily tasks.

Reishi is what I consider the calming mushroom. It works beautifully in the evening to settle your nervous system, lower nighttime cortisol, and help your body shift into rest-and-repair mode.[9] If your mind is constantly spinning when your head hits the pillow or you wake up at 2:00 a.m. unable to shut your brain off, reishi can be a game changer. It gently coaxes your stress response toward balance.

Licorice root is one supplement that necessitates extreme caution. It is incredibly helpful for people with low cortisol because it extends the half-life of cortisol and helps your body maintain a more stable rhythm.[10] But it should NOT be used in anyone with high cortisol. If your cortisol is already elevated, licorice will make things worse, not better. This is why I say you should never just throw an adrenal supplement at yourself willy-nilly. You have to know what your cortisol pattern looks like from proper testing before adding anything targeted, or you can accidentally push your body further out of balance.

Meditation and Breath Work
Meditation and breath work can shift your nervous system out of fight-or-flight mode and into a state where healing is possible. I personally believe that breath work is one of the best ways to calm your nervous system, and you don't need an hour of meditation to get results. Just a few minutes of intentional breathing can make a difference and lower your cortisol level, especially at night when your brain won't shut off.

One of my favorite techniques is box breathing: Inhale for four counts, hold for four, exhale for four, hold for four, and repeat. It sounds simple, but it works.

Blue Light Blocking
Too much blue light from screens is one of the sneakiest hormone disruptors out there. While you're staring at your phone, laptop, or TV in the evening, that blue light is telling your brain it's daytime. Your body needs the signal that it's dark so it can make melatonin, the hormone that counters cortisol and helps you fall and remain asleep. Melatonin and

cortisol have an inverse relationship, meaning that when one is high, the other is typically low, and this balance is important for regulating circadian rhythms and sleep.

If your melatonin is blocked, your circadian rhythms go off track, and instead of winding down at night, your body pumps out more cortisol. Over time, a constantly elevated cortisol level doesn't just throw off your sleep habits, it affects your thyroid, too.

The good news is that this is an easy fix to make. At sunset, throw on a pair of blue light–blocking glasses and set your screens to night mode. You don't have to give up technology or sit around by candlelight, you just need to stop signaling your brain that it's noon when it's really 9:00 p.m. This will help restore normal cortisol patterns and better sleep, which will ensure that your thyroid has the environment it needs to function properly.

· · ·

Finding strategies for coping with stress is worth the effort because when you calm your body's stress response, you create a physiological environment in which your thyroid can do what it was meant to do. And you won't just feel better—you'll be happier, too.

Biohacking Breakthroughs: GLPs and Other Strategies to Supercharge Your Thyroid Health

---

You can't outbiohack a wrecked thyroid that isn't being treated properly. No amount of fancy devices, red light panels, or supplements is going to make up for a lack of thyroid hormones if your levels are at rock bottom. But once you have the basics in place—proper labs, the right medication, good nutrition, and stress management—you can take advantage of powerful tools that will help your thyroid function better, reduce inflammation, and support your energy. Those tools can be grouped together in a category called "biohacking."

These days, when you hear the word *biohacking*, it's easy to feel overwhelmed. Everywhere you turn, there's some doctor or influencer or longevity guru telling you about the latest cool thing you should be doing to be truly healthy. I, too, used to feel the pressure of having to do it all: forty-five minutes in the sauna, fifteen minutes in the cold plunge, twenty minutes of meditating, fifteen minutes of breath work, twenty minutes in front of the red light, five thousand different supplements, lying on a pulsed electronic magnetic field (PEMF) mat, running at different frequencies, more breath work, more meditation, hyperbaric oxygen, vagus nerve stimulation—honestly, it felt like a full-time job just trying to optimize my health. If that's what you think biohacking is, you're never going to do it.

Biohacking is really just the art and science of making small, intentional tweaks beyond baseline medication so that your body works better. Think of it as stacking the deck in your favor. These are little, strategic interventions that will move the needle so you're not just surviving, you're thriving. The good news is that you don't have to be billionaire biohacker Brian Johnson to biohack your thyroid and see results. You don't need tens of thousands of dollars, and you don't need to spend five hours a day jumping from one gadget to the next. These tools and techniques are available to anyone and can bolster everything you're already doing with optimized medication and a smartly modified lifestyle.

And in this case, we're being focused: We're talking about biohacks that will specifically benefit your thyroid.

GLPs

One of the most exciting biohacks for thyroid has emerged in recent years almost by accident: GLP-1s, the popular and controversial weight loss drugs that include Ozempic, Wegovy, and Mounjaro, have turned out to have effects and benefits far beyond the glucose-lowering, insulin-correcting, appetite-suppressing activity for which they were developed. It turns out that GLP-1s' impact on metabolism leads to lower bodywide inflammation, particularly inflammation in the brain,[1] and that this may directly affect your TSH level, slightly improving thyroid function. This may also potentially lower thyroid antibodies, because when inflammation in the body goes down, antibodies often follow. Whatever the exact mechanism of action, I have witnessed these effects among patients in my practice and corroborated them through labs and thyroid panels. GLP-1s, in microdose form, are showing promise as an incredible tool for supporting thyroid health—when used in conjunction with proper thyroid medication, of course.

I'll admit that when glucagon-like peptide-1 receptor agonists (GLP-1s) first came out, I lovingly dubbed them the Beverly Hills soccer mom weight loss drug of choice. Stories abounded about "Ozempic face" and people losing so much weight that they looked skeletal—and GLP-1s were either glorified or demonized with very little in between. But in my view, it's in this gray zone that the potential of GLP-1s, and the next generations of GLP-2s, GLP-3s, and GLP-4s, really lies.

All GLPs work by mimicking hormones that your gut naturally produces, such as glucagon-like peptide-1. They were originally developed to treat type 2 diabetes by helping regulate blood sugar, which they do by increasing insulin secretion, slowing down gastric emptying, and reducing appetite. They are truly breakthrough medications, in my opinion. But like most other drugs, whether they are a poison or a cure depends on the dose. We've all read the horror stories of otherwise healthy people who took high doses of GLP-1s intended for diabetics and developed severe side effects including muscle wasting, gastroparesis, and irritable bowel syndrome (IBS). Or the diabetic patients who kept increasing their doses unnecessarily, resulting in severe side effects. The truth is that standard doses are meant for individuals with advanced metabolic disease, not someone simply looking to lose ten pounds.

That's when the influencers and fearmongers came onto the scene, scaring people away from these medications using broad-brush claims and painting them as dangerous shortcuts. But while some people are fretting about the side effects, others like Dr. Tyna Moore, Dr. Gus Vickery, and I are saying, "Hold on, let's look at the bigger picture." There's a right way to use GLPs. And when used correctly, the results are nothing short of phenomenal.

Enter microdosing.

Microdosing GLPs means using a fraction of what a conventional doctor might prescribe for someone with type 2 diabetes. We're talking 70 to 90 percent less than the standard diabetic protocol. We are finding that at such a low dose, the benefits of GLPs mostly remain, while the side effects vanish. And it turns out that at these lower doses, there can be real benefits for the thyroid. Here's what I see.

1. **Improved metabolic health.** Even at low doses, GLPs support insulin sensitivity and can help with blood sugar stabilization and fat loss. Microdosing is *not* a weight loss fix, however. It's supporting your

metabolism, not jacking it through the roof. You can't eat garbage and skip the gym; you still have to do your part. However, GLPs at low doses can still improve insulin resistance and thereby reduce the chronic bodywide inflammation that exacerbates Hashimoto's and impedes thyroid function.

When one of our patients decides to start a GLP, whether it is a standard dose for weight loss or a microdose for inflammation, there is a nonnegotiable agreement. And it is this: You are pledging to do your part. If you take this medication, you will eat protein like it is your second job. You will lift something heavy on a regular basis and protect your muscle mass as if your life depends on it, because in the long run . . . it does. You will do resistance training in some form, week after week, no excuses. You will treat your body with intention.

Because here's the truth: If you don't, this medication will be a waste of your money and our time. GLPs are not magic. They are a tool, and like any tool, they work only when you use them alongside the right habits.

Microdosing helps because it supports insulin sensitivity without wiping out appetite and muscle. It lets your metabolism breathe a little. And when your thyroid is optimized, your body responds even better.

2. **Cardiovascular protection.** People always bring up the cardiovascular protection that comes with GLPs as though it is in its own separate category, but it actually ties right back to your thyroid. When your thyroid function is low, everything that impacts your heart starts sliding in the wrong direction. Your cholesterol levels go up, your blood pressure inches up, your blood sugar becomes harder to manage, and your inflammation climbs. That combination alone increases cardiovascular risk long before you feel it.

When someone uses a GLP-1 in a microdose and suddenly their blood sugar is steadier, their inflammation calms down, and they start losing body fat instead of muscle, that of course helps the heart. But if your thyroid is also fully optimized, the cardiovascular benefits from the GLP-1 will be even more dramatic: You'll see changes in your labs, in your cholesterol levels, and even in how your heart feels when you wake up in the morning.[2]

3. **Enhanced liver function.** In addition to reducing overall inflammation, GLPs reduce fat buildup in the liver, leading to a better environment for liver cells to function in.[3] When the liver is healthy, T4 to T3 conversion improves along with overall metabolism.

4. **Better brain function and mental health.** We've talked about the brain fog and mood issues that can accompany thyroid dysfunction, and it turns out that microdosing GLPs can have neuroprotective effects. By reducing inflammation in the brain, these small doses can lead to improvements in ADHD symptoms, mood stabilization, and reduced frequency of migraines.[4] I had a patient, Lana, who started a microdose of a GLP for its metabolic and thyroid benefits. But within days, she noticed that her mood had lifted and her panic attacks had disappeared. She ultimately stopped needing to take Xanax entirely. That's the power of reducing neuroinflammation.

5. **Lower thyroid-stimulating hormone (TSH) levels.** For me, the proof of any legitimate impact on the thyroid is: Can we measure it in thyroid labs? In the case of GLPs, the answer is yes. Over time, I am consistently seeing a reduction in TSH levels in patients who are using microdoses of GLPs to support their thyroid. Remember, the higher your TSH level, the harder your brain has to work to get your thyroid to respond. But it appears as though GLPs, through reducing brain inflammation, also improve the communication among the hypothalamus, pituitary, and thyroid along the HPT axis, resulting in a better thyroid response.

. . .

At this time, there are no studies showing a direct correlation between using GLPs and improvements in free T3 or reverse T3. But I believe they're coming, and in my own practice, we've seen some compelling trends. I've had numerous patients who, after starting a microdose of GLP-1, were able to reduce their T3 medication by as much as 25 to 50 mg per day. Even I have been able to reduce my own T3 medication when on a GLP-1, going from 150 mcg per day down to 100 mcg daily with no hypothyroid symptoms. In the past when I played around with lowering my T3 dose, *any* drop in T3 would cause the weight to rapidly come back on, and my whole body would be inflamed and angry. For the first time in twenty-five years, I've stayed optimal even with a lower T3 dose.

Now, I've said it before and I'll say it again: Your goal is not to be on the lowest possible dose of thyroid medication. That's not the point. There's no gold star given out to people on the lowest dose of thyroid medication. We replace hormones because our body's not making them. I don't care what I'm on and I don't care what you're on, as long as it works and you get your life back. *But* there are some perks to being on a lower dose of T3 medication—for example, as I talked about in the chapter on T2, when T3 boosts your metabolism, it doesn't discriminate between burning fat and burning muscle, whereas T2 burns fat and leaves muscle alone. So if you can drop your T3 slightly and retain your sexy, lean muscle while still feeling optimized and amazing, that's a win.

That's why I believe that GLPs, when microdosed properly, are more than a trendy biohacking tool. They may well become a cornerstone of thyroid treatment in the years ahead, because the science around them is advancing every day, and we are just getting started. The biggest con with microdosing GLPs is . . . their cost. They are expensive, and at the time of this writing, most insurance companies will not cover them unless you meet strict criteria, such as a diagnosis of type 2 diabetes or a body mass index (BMI) of over 30 with related health conditions. The cost can range from several hundred to even a few thousand dollars a month, depending on the source and the compound. For some people, it is a worthwhile investment; for others, it's out of reach.

The other thing I want to make clear is that GLPs, on their own, are not a miracle drug. If your thyroid is tanked, your hormones are wrecked, your reverse T3 is sky-high, and your inflammation is off the charts, GLPs will not override that. I don't care how aggressive your dose is or how many influencers say it worked for them, if you haven't fixed the thyroid, these peptides won't do a thing.

My patient Tamara is one of the best examples of this. She came to me initially not for thyroid help but because she had been diagnosed with type 2 diabetes. She was carrying an extra 150 pounds, and she had been prescribed a GLP-1 medication (Ozempic) by her doctor, but it wasn't working. Her blood sugar level had not improved, and the weight hadn't budged.

When we ran new labs, we discovered that she was in a deep hypothyroid state. Her T3 was low, her reverse T3 was high, and she wasn't on any sort of hormone replacement therapy, even though she was well into menopause. Once we addressed her thyroid and optimized her hormones, everything clicked. The GLP-1 started doing its job, her metabolism began responding, her inflammation dropped, and her body began working for her and not against her. Tamara has now fully reversed her type 2 diabetes and lost more than a hundred pounds.

That is why I always caution people that GLPs are remarkable in many ways, but if your thyroid is dragging and your other hormones are flatlined due to perimenopause or menopause, they won't do what they are designed to do. You first need to get the other pieces of the puzzle into place. Then, when you are stable and optimized, adding a GLP can take your thyroid function and your overall health to the next level.

Who Should *Not* Use GLPs, Even in Microdose Form

While GLP-1s have a good safety profile and microdosing is generally well tolerated, there are still a few hard stops. If you have a personal or family history of medullary thyroid carcinoma (MTC) or multiple endocrine neoplasia syndrome type 2 (MEN 2), GLP receptor agonists may not be for you. These medications come with a black box warning about these conditions, and while the data about them is limited to animal studies, it's not something to take lightly. However, it's important to note that the black box warning on GLP-1s was the result of rodent studies in which the doses used were much higher than what a human would take, roughly twenty times as high as the maximum human dose. At that extreme level, the rodents developed C cell (cells that are responsible for the growth of thyroid cancer) changes in the thyroid, which then got translated into the warning.

Here is the important thing to remember: Humans do not have the same density of C cells that those rodents had, and our C cells do not respond to GLPs the same way. We have years of real-world human data now, and there has been no documented increase in medullary thyroid carcinoma in people taking normal therapeutic doses of GLPs. So yes, the warning is technically there, but the conditions under which that warning originated do not match real human use at all.

Similarly, if you have a history of disordered eating such as anorexia, bulimia, or orthorexia, there is the potential for even the slightest food aversion or appetite suppression to trigger restrictive tendencies, even at a microdosed level. If this has been an issue for you in the past, you need to move forward with GLPs with careful awareness and oversight.

Red Light Therapy

I'll be honest with you: Even though I live and breathe functional medicine, it seemed a little far-fetched to me that shining a red light on your neck could help your thyroid heal. I was hugely skeptical. Really? Just light?

I went down the research rabbit hole (as I so often do) looking for proof to contradict its effectiveness. I looked high and low for a study that said it didn't work, and I couldn't find one. Every study I found, including a 2023 study published in the *Journal of Personalized Medicine*, showed that red light therapy has a positive impact on thyroid health, sometimes even lowering thyroid antibodies.[5]

You've probably seen it all over Instagram by now, but here's how it works: Red light therapy is a form of low-level laser therapy that uses specific wavelengths of red and near-infrared light to promote healing and improve cellular function. Red light tends to work more on the surface of the body, boosting circulation, calming inflammation, and helping with skin and tissue repair.[6] Near-infrared light goes deeper. It can actually reach your thyroid gland and even stimulate the mitochondria, those little energy factories inside your cells.

That deeper penetration is why near-infrared light is especially powerful for thyroid health. When the light hits the thyroid, it interacts with an enzyme in your mitochondria called cytochrome c oxidase, which stimulates them to make energy faster and more efficiently.[7] When thyroid cells have more energy, they work better, and there are improvements in hormone output.

The best part? You don't need a giant clinical setup to get the benefits. There are plenty of at-home panels and handheld devices now that use the right therapeutic wavelengths. Even a few minutes a day with the light directed at your thyroid area can start making a difference. Red light therapy feeds your mitochondria, reduces inflammation, and helps your thyroid make and use hormones more effectively. This is one of the most promising nondrug tools we have for supporting thyroid health.

Cold Therapy

Cold exposure isn't just for hardcore Wim Hof types sitting in an ice-covered river. Even brief cold exposure, such as a cold shower or a quick ice bath, has real benefits. When your body hits the cold water, brown fat—the good kind of fat that burns energy to keep you warm—is activated. The more active your brown fat is, the more calories you burn and the more you stoke your basal metabolic rate.

Cold also stimulates your vagus nerve, helping your body calm down, recover faster from stress, and return to a steadier, more resilient state.[8] The vagus nerve extends from your brain stem to your abdomen, and it regulates your body's automatic functions, such as breathing, heart rate, and digestion. Crucially, it works in opposition to the sympathetic nervous system, which activates your body's fight-or-flight response. Activating the vagus nerve shifts you out of fight-or-flight mode and into a calmer state, helping bring down your cortisol level and improving your resilience to stress. If you partake in cold exposure, you might notice that you sleep better, recover faster after workouts, or feel more grounded overall. As you lower your cortisol level and your body's stress response, you improve your thyroid's overall environment.

Cold exposure does not have to be extreme to work. You are not trying to shock your system into panic mode; instead you are training your body to adapt. For good thyroid health, moderation is key. A simple way to start is finishing your normal shower with thirty seconds of cold water. If you tolerate that well, you can build up to a minute or two of cold water or try a cold plunge a couple of times a week. Some people even find that it helps with mood and mental clarity. That blast of cold water wakes you up, improves your circulation, lowers your inflammation, and gets your brain firing.

Sauna and Heat Therapy

Heat exposure, such as in an infrared sauna, is one of my favorite tools to support good thyroid and hormone health. When you sit in the heat, your body starts to sweat, and sweating is a primary way of getting rid of toxins. Heavy metals, plastics, pesticides, and all the other endocrine disruptors stored up in your fat tissue start to move out. You lighten the toxic load on your body every time you sweat them out.

A sauna also improves your circulation and gets your blood moving, bringing more oxygen and nutrients to your tissues. The heat also supports your lymphatic system, the part of your immune system that functions as your body's drainage system. A sluggish lymph system can mean persistent inflammation, fatigue, and slower healing because your body can't effectively clear waste. A healthy lymph system lowers inflammation, which is especially important if you are struggling with thyroid-related autoimmunity.

In addition to improving lymphatic circulation, sauna sessions can lower your cortisol level, boost your relaxation, and give you that "ahh" reset feeling. You might even sleep better after heat exposure.

I know that not everyone has access to an infrared sauna. You can still get some of the benefits with a hot bath. Toss in Epsom salts to add magnesium, which relaxes your muscles, supports detoxification, and calms your nervous system. It may not be the same as an infrared sauna, but it will still help your body release toxins, reduce stress, and support recovery.

Aim for a few sessions per week, and think of it as part of your thyroid care routine. Just as lifting weights builds strength and cold exposure builds resilience, heat exposure helps your body let go of what is weighing it down.

Pulsed Electromagnetic Field (PEMF) Therapy

Pulsed electromagnetic field therapy (PEMF) is like a recharge for your cells. You lie down on a mat that generates low-frequency electromagnetic pulses that penetrate your body. Our cells naturally use electrical signals to carry out different functions, but stress, illness, or injury can cause their electrical charge to drop, impeding their ability to exchange nutrients or remove waste. A PEMF mat acts like a battery charger, enhancing cellular function and activity, improving circulation, and lowering inflammation. It also spurs your mitochondria to work better and generate more energy.[9] If you're tired all the time, even when you're getting enough sleep, PEMF therapy can help.

PEMF therapy is simple. You just lie on a mat for ten to twenty minutes while you're reading, watching TV, or winding down. I keep mine on the couch, so I'll use it at night while I'm answering emails or catching up on a show. It's not flashy or dramatic, you don't feel "zapped" or anything like that, but it gives your body extra support. Over time, you will notice better energy, recovery, and metabolic function.

Exposure to Morning Light

This is such an overlooked, easy to do, and enjoyable biohack. Getting natural light in your eyes within thirty to sixty minutes of waking sets your circadian rhythm, your body's internal clock. When that clock is properly set, your cortisol level rises exactly when it should, in the morning, giving you energy, and your whole day flows more smoothly.

Morning light also boosts dopamine, the neurotransmitter that drives motivation and focus. You know those mornings when you feel as though you just cannot get going no matter how much coffee you drink? That is often a circadian issue, not a caffeine one.

I live in Iowa, and in December, the sun doesn't come up until 7:00 a.m. I'm up at six, and at that hour, it's about 32 degrees outside. So no, I'm not stepping outside in the freezing dark or doing sunrise yoga in a parka. But I still do what I can. Even a few minutes standing by a window or using a light therapy lamp makes a difference.

That said, nothing beats sunlight. Even on a cloudy day, the light outside is ten to a hundred times more powerful for your brain and hormones than anything indoors. If you can bundle up and go outside for five to ten minutes with your morning coffee, walk the dog, or just stand in the daylight, your thyroid and your energy level will thank you.

Grounding

Getting your bare feet on the earth, also called grounding or earthing, is another simple way to calm your body. When your skin connects with the ground, you absorb electrons from the earth that help lower inflammation and regulate your nervous system.[10] Grounding has been shown to lower cortisol and improve sleep, which directly support thyroid function.

You don't need to spend hours to make it work. Even ten minutes a day barefoot in your yard, at a park, or in the dirt of your garden is enough to start noticing the benefits. And when you can stack it with morning sunlight, you get the best of both worlds. Light helps set your circadian rhythm, while grounding brings your stress response down. Together, they impact your inflammation and hormone balance.

When the weather is warm, I take my coffee outside, stand in the grass, and get light and grounding in at the same time. On cold mornings, I lean on light therapy inside and catch up on grounding later in the day. The point is, do what you can.

. . .

Biohacking doesn't necessarily mean using flashy gadgets or living in a lab; it's simply about pulling from both modern science and old-school wisdom to create the kind of environment in which your thyroid can thrive.

I recommend that you pick one or two of these strategies to start with. If you are optimized and stable on your thyroid meds, talk to your doctor about GLPs. Layer these different strategies on slowly, see how your body responds, and keep building from there. This is not about being perfect; it's about stacking wins and making progress.

When you pair smart biohacks with the right medication, solid nutrition, and a positive mindset, everything shifts. That's when you stop just getting by and finally start living. And remember this: Your thyroid doesn't have the final word. You do.

It All Comes Down to You

You've made it this far. You've read every page, story, and science-backed suggestion I've made. You always knew you weren't broken, lazy, crazy, or destined to feel like you do forever.

This is the moment when you decide what comes next. You can go back to the old way of doing things. You can keep accepting half-assed answers and quick dismissals, the tired lines about eating less and moving more, the prescriptions that never address the root cause. You can keep hoping the next diet or the next detox will finally be the thing that works.

Or you can take a different path. You can become the CEO of your own health. You can demand the labs that will tell you the truth. You can work with practitioners who hear you, who respect you, who treat you like a partner rather than a problem to be managed. You can honor your body for every signal it sends you, every symptom that is never random but is trying to show you where to look.

Most important, you can imagine the life waiting for you on the other side of all this: waking up with energy and a clear head, feeling rested and ready to take on your day; looking in the mirror and seeing your face bright, your skin healthy, your hair growing back, your confidence returning; having a glass of wine or a piece of cake at a friend's birthday and not having to worry about the extra pounds you'll have to take off the next day; feeling present in your relationships, connected to your purpose, alive in your own skin.

It's what can happen when you optimize your thyroid and other hormones. It's what can happen when you refuse to settle for less than the full expression of your health. The way forward is not always simple. It requires persistence. It also requires asking better questions. You need to show up for yourself again and again, even when you feel discouraged. But I can assure you: You are worth every ounce of effort it takes to get there.

If you take away one thing from this book, let it be this: Your future is not written in the labs that said you were normal or the doctors who shrugged off your symptoms. Your story does not end with fatigue, brain fog, weight gain, and the hollow ache of wondering what happened to you. Your story is still being written. And it all comes down to you.

Today is the day you decide to choose hope over helplessness, action over avoidance, and truth over trends. Today is the day you become the advocate you have always needed. I'm right here, cheering you on.

Take a deep breath. Stand a little taller. This is just the beginning. The journey that began when you picked up this book is the one that will lead you back to you.

Acknowledgments

To my support system, my husband, Jason. You are my rock, my anchor, and my safe place. You've encouraged me to push past my limits, to grow, and to believe in myself when doubt crept in. You stood by me through my cancer journey, holding me up when I felt like falling, reminding me that I was stronger than the storm. Without you, I wouldn't be here, and this book would not exist. Your love, patience, and unwavering support have carried me through the hardest days and given me the strength to keep going. This is as much yours as it is mine.

To my publisher, Simon & Schuster, my agent, Beth Davey, and my editors, Patti Hall and Ann Campbell—thank you for taking what lived only in my head and helping me shape it into something real, powerful, and ready for the women who need it most. You didn't just bring a book to life; you helped refine my voice without softening it, sharpen the message without diluting the truth, and guide this work from raw idea to finished pages that can finally reach millions. Your belief in this message, your patience in the process, and your commitment to honoring my voice made this possible. Without each of you, this book would still be a vision instead of a lifeline in the hands of the people it was written for.

To my team, the ones who run just as hard and just as fast as I do. You don't flinch when the vision gets bigger or the pace gets intense. You rise, adapt, and execute with heart, precision, and purpose. Because of you, this work doesn't stall. It scales. You carry the mission when the days are long, protect the standard when it would be easier to cut corners, and show up every day knowing that what we do changes lives. Together, we are building something that reaches far beyond any one of us, and because of your commitment, grit, and belief in this mission, we get to help millions of women reclaim their health, their power, and their lives. This impact is possible because of you.

And a special thank-you to my CMO, Jill Bunny. You have been by my side through the frustration, the tears, and the laughter, and you are a cornerstone of bringing this book into the world. You work on this mission with the same intensity, care, and commitment that I do, and your belief in this message never wavers. Having walked your own thyroid cancer journey, you deeply understand what's at stake when women are dismissed or misinformed about their health. Your passion for creating a movement where women wake up, advocate for themselves, and take control of their bodies has shaped this work in ways I could never put into words. This book carries your heart, your grit, and your unwavering dedication to women everywhere.

Notes

Introduction

1. Wyne, K, L. Nair, C. Schneiderman, et al., "Hypothyroidism Prevalence in the United States: A Retrospective Study Combining National Health and Nutrition Examination Survey and Claims Data, 2009–2019," *Journal of the Endocrine Society* 7 (2022), doi.org/10.1210/jendso/bvac172.
2. Journy, N., M. Bernier, M. Doody, et al, "Hyperthyroidism, Hypothyroidism, and Cause-Specific Mortality in a Large Cohort of Women," *Thyroid* 27, no. 8 (2017), doi.org/10.1089/thy.2017.0063.

Chapter 1: Listen to Your Body, That's Your Thyroid Talking

1. Antonelli, A., P. Fallahi, S. Ferrari, et al., "3,5-diiodo-L-thyronine Increases Resting Metabolic Rate and Reduces Body Weight without Undesirable Side Effects," *Journal of Biological Regulators and Homeostatic Agents* 25, no. 4 (2011): 655–60, www.europepmc.org/article/med/22217997; and Lombardi, A., R. Senese, R. D. Matteis, et al., "3,5-diiodo-lthyronine Activates Brown Adipose Tissue Thermogenesis in Hypothyroid Rats," *PLOS One* 10, no. 2 (2015), doi.org/10.1371/journal.pone.0116498.
2. Mullur, R., Y. Liu, and G. Brent, "Thyroid Hormone Regulation of Metabolism," *Physiological Reviews* 94, no. 2 (2014): 355–82, doi.org/10.1152/physrev.00030.2013.
3. Yau, W. and P. Yen, "Thermogenesis in Adipose Tissue Activated by Thyroid Hormone," *International Journal of Molecular Sciences* 21, no. 8 (2020), doi.org/10.3390/ijms21083020.
4. Forini, F., V. Lionetti, H. Ardehali, et al., "Early Long-term l-t3 Replacement Rescues Mitochondria and Prevents Ischemic Cardiac Remodeling in Rats," *Journal of Cellular and Molecular Medicine* 15, no. 3 (2010): 514–24, doi.org/10.1111/j.1582-4934.2010.01014.x.
5. Nomura, S., C. S. Pittman, J. B. Chambers, et al., Reduced Peripheral Conversion of Thyroxine to Triiodothyronine in Patients with Hepatic Cirrhosis," *Journal of Clinical Investigation* 56, no. 3 (1975): 643–52, doi.org/10.1172/jci108134.
6. Silberman, D., M. Wald, and A. Genaro, "Effects of Chronic Mild Stress on Lymphocyte Proliferative Response. Participation of Serum Thyroid Hormones and Corticosterone," *International Immunopharmacology* 2, no. 4 (2002): 487–97, doi.org/10.1016/s1567-5769(01)00190-4; Mancini, A., C. Di Segni, S. Raimondo, et al., "Thyroid Hormones, Oxidative Stress, and Inflammation," *Mediators of Inflammation* (2016), doi.org/10.1155/2016/6757154; Agnihothri, R., A. Courville, J. Linderman, et al., "Moderate Weight Loss Is Sufficient to Affect Thyroid Hormone Homeostasis and Inhibit Its Peripheral Conversion," *Thyroid* 24, no. 1 (2014): 19–26, doi.org/10.1089/thy.2013.0055; and Fisher, D. "Physiological Variations in Thyroid Hormones: Physiological and Pathophysiological Considerations," *Clinical Chemistry* 42, no. 1 (1996): 135–39, doi.org/10.1093/clinchem/42.1.135.
7. Beckett, G., S. Beddows, P. Morrice, et al., "Inhibition of Hepatic Deiodination of Thyroxine Is Caused by Selenium Deficiency in Rats," *Biochemical Journal* 248, no. 2 (1987):

443–47, doi.org/10.1042/bj2480443; Krishnamurthy, H., S. Reddy, V. Jayaraman, et al., "Effect of Micronutrients on Thyroid Parameters," *Journal of Thyroid Research* (2021), doi .org/10.1155/2021/1865483; and Kabadi, U., B. Premachandra, and M. Maayan, "Low Serum 3, 5, 3'-triiodothyronine (T3) and raised 3, 3', 5'-triidothyronine (Reverse T3 or RT3) in Diabetes Mellitus: Normalization on Improvement in Hyperglycemia," *Acta Diabetologia Latina* 19 (1982): 233–42, doi.org/10.1007/bf02624683.

Chapter 2: Your Body's Loudest Thyroid Distress Signals

1. Lee, M. and J. Kim, J., "The Pathophysiology of Visceral Adipose Tissues in Cardiometabolic Diseases," *Biochemical Pharmacology* 222 (2024), doi.org/10.1016/j.bcp.2024.116116; Sun, Y., X. Shan, M. Li, et al., "Autoimmune Mechanisms and Inflammation in Obesity-Associated Type 2 Diabetes, Atherosclerosis, and Non-alcoholic Fatty Liver Disease," *Functional & Integrative Genomics* 25 (2025), doi.org/10.1007/s10142-025-01587-0; and Luo, J., Y. Wang, J. Mao, et al., "Features, Functions, and Associated Diseases of Visceral and Ectopic Fat: A Comprehensive Review," *Obesity* 33, no. 5 (2025): 825–38, doi.org/10.1002 /oby.24239.

2. Lombardi, A., R. Senese, R. D. Matteis, et al., "3,5-diiodo-l-thyronine Activates Brown Adipose Tissue Thermogenesis in Hypothyroid Rats," *PLOS One* 10, no. 2 (2015), doi.org/10.1371 /journal.pone.0116498.

3. Chondronikola, M., F. Volpi, E. B.rsheim, et al., "Brown Adipose Tissue Improves Whole-Body Glucose Homeostasis and Insulin Sensitivity in Humans," *Diabetes* 63, no. 12 (2014): 4089–99, doi.org/10.2337/db14-0746.

4. Sędzikowska, A. and L. Szablewski, "Insulin and Insulin Resistance in Alzheimer's Disease," *International Journal of Molecular Sciences* 22, no. 18 (2021), doi.org/10.3390 /ijms22189987.

5. Kraemer, W., N. Ratamess, W. Hymer, et al., "Growth Hormone(s), Testosterone, Insulin-Like Growth Factors, and Cortisol: Roles and Integration for Cellular Development and Growth with Exercise," *Frontiers in Endocrinology* 11 (2020), doi.org/10.3389/fendo.2020.00033; and Salehian, B., and K. Kejriwal, "Glucocorticoid-induced Muscle Atrophy: Mechanisms and Therapeutic Strategies," *Endocrine Practice* 5, no. 5 (1999): 277–81, doi.org/10.4158 /ep.5.5.277.

6. Liu, S., J. Ma, L. Zhang, et al., "Circulating Leptin Levels in Thyroid Dysfunction: A Systematic Review and Meta-Analysis." *BMC Endocrine Disorders* 25 (2025), doi.org/10.1186/s12902 -025-01943-y.

7. Michael Powell, *Diagnosis and Treatment of Human Dormancy Syndrome*, U.S. Patent 7,648,704, filed October 8, 2007, and issued January 19, 2010, www.patents.google.com /patent/US7288257B2/en.

8. Rajasundaram, S., R. Rahman, B. Woolf, et al., "Morning Cortisol and Circulating Inflammatory Cytokine Levels: A Mendelian Randomisation Study," *Genes* 13, no. 1 (2022), doi.org /10.3390/genes13010116.

9. Vyunytska, L., T. Yuzvenko, T. Dashuk, et al., "Stress-induced Urgent Conditions in Endocrinology," *International Journal of Endocrinology (Ukraine)* 20, no.1 (2024), doi .org/10.22141/2224-0721.20.1.2024.1360; and Javid, M., S. U. Khan, M. Akram, et al., "Higher Cortisol Level and Reduced Circulating Triiodothyronine in Patients with Cardiovascular Diseases: A Case-Control Study," *JRSM Cardiovascular Disease* (2025), www.pubmed.ncbi .nlm.nih.gov/40386768/.

10. Daher R, T. Yazbeck, J. B. Jaoude, et al., "Consequences of Dysthyroidism on the Digestive Tract and Viscera," *World Journal of Gastroenterology* 15, no. 23 (2009): 2834–38, doi:10.3748 /wjg.15.2834.

11. Dai, Y., Y. Tai, Y. Chang, et al., "Bidirectional Association Between Alopecia Areata and Thyroid Diseases: A Nationwide Population-Based Cohort Study," *Archives of Dermatological Research* 313 (2020): 339–46, doi.org/10.1007/s00403-020-02109-7.

12. Martin, J. and P. Sarkar, "Nongenomic Roles of Thyroid Hormones and Their Derivatives in Adult Brain: Are These Compounds Putative Neurotransmitters?" *Frontiers in Endocrinology* 14 (2023), doi.org/10.3389/fendo.2023.1210540.

13. Bode, H., B. Ivens, T, Bschor, et al., "Association of Hypothyroidism and Clinical Depression: A Systematic Review and Meta-analysis," *JAMA Psychiatry* 78, no. 12 (2021), doi.org/10.1001/jamapsychiatry.2021.2506.

14. Maddox, S., O. Ponomareva, C. Zaleski, et al., "Evidence for Thyroid Hormone Regulation of Amygdala-Dependent Fear-Relevant Memory and Plasticity," *Molecular Psychiatry* 30 (2024): 201–12, doi.org/10.1038/s41380-024-02679-2; and Bárez-López, S., A. Montero-Pedrazuela, D. Bosch-García, et al., "Increased Anxiety and Fear Memory in Adult Mice Lacking Type 2 Deiodinase," *Psychoneuroendocrinology* 84 (2017): 51–60, doi.org/10.1016/j.psyneuen.2017.06.013.

15. Bernardes, B., M. De Oliveira Borba, S. Moreira, et al., "Relationship Between Mood Disorders and Thyroid Changes," *Brazilian Journal of Implantology and Health Sciences* 6 no. 2 (2024), doi.org/10.36557/2674-8169.2024v6n2p2241-2256; and Lorentzen, R., J. Kjaer, S. Stergaard, et al., "Thyroid Hormone Treatment in the Management of Treatment-Resistant Unipolar Depression: A Systematic Review and Meta-analysis," *Acta Psychiatrica Scandinavica* 141, no. 4 (2020), doi.org/10.1111/acps.13154.

16. Chuang, S., Y. Chen, S. Huang, et al., "Association Between Adhesive Capsulitis and Thyroid Disease: A Meta-Analysis," *Journal of Shoulder and Elbow Surgery* 32, no. 6 (2023): 1314–22, doi.org/10.1016/j.jse.2023.01.033.

17. Meshram, K., A. Rawekar, A. Meshram, et al., "Nerve Conduction Study in Early Diagnosed Cases of Hypothyroidism in Central India," *Indian Journal of Forensic Medicine & Toxicology* 14, no. 4 (2020), doi.org/10.37506/ijfmt.v14i4.12760.

18. Di Vincenzo, F., A. Del Gaudio, V. Petito, et al., "Gut Microbiota, Intestinal Permeability, and Systemic Inflammation: A Narrative Review," *Internal and Emergency Medicine* 19 (2023): 275–93, doi.org/10.1007/s11739-023-03374-w.

19. Değirmenci, P., C. Kirmaz, D. Oz, et al., "Allergic Rhinitis and Its Relationship with Autoimmune Thyroid Diseases," *American Journal of Rhinology & Allergy* 29 (2015): 257–61, doi.org/10.2500/ajra.2015.29.4189.

20. Nowaczewska, M., M. Straburzynski, G. Meder, et al., "The Relationship Between Migraine and Hashimoto's Thyroiditis: A Single Center Experience," *Frontiers in Neurology* 15 (2024), doi.org/10.3389/fneur.2024.1370530.

21. Yamakawa, H., T. Kato, J. Noh, et al., "Thyroid Hormone Plays an Important Role in Cardiac Function: From Bench to Bedside," *Frontiers in Physiology* 12 (2021), doi.org/10.3389/fphys.2021.606931.

22. Nowaczewska, Straburzynski, Meder, et al., "The Relationship Between Migraine and Hashimoto's Thyroiditis."

Chapter 3: How Did I Get Here?

1. Fasano, A., "Leaky Gut and Autoimmune Diseases," *Clinical Reviews in Allergy & Immunology* 42 (2012): 71–78, www.springer.com/article/10.1007/s12016-011-8291-x.

2. Raetz, C. R. and C. Whitfield, "Lipopolysaccharide Endotoxins," *Annual Review of Biochemistry* 71 (2002), www.pubmed.ncbi.nlm.nih.gov/12045108.

3. Romano, R., J. De Oliveira, V. De Oliveira, et al., "Could Glyphosate and Glyphosate-Based Herbicides Be Associated with Increased Thyroid Diseases Worldwide?" *Frontiers in Endocrinology* 12 (2021), doi.org/10.3389/fendo.2021.627167; and Mazuryk, J., K. Klepacka, W. Kutner, et al., "Glyphosate: Hepatotoxicity, Nephrotoxicity, Hemotoxicity, Carcinogenicity, and Clinical Cases of Endocrine, Reproductive, Cardiovascular, and Pulmonary System Intoxication," *ACS Pharmacology & Translational Science* 7, no. 5 (2024):1205–36, doi.org/10.1021/acsptsci.4c00046.

4. Kongtip, P., N. Nankongnab, R. Pundee, et al., "Acute Changes in Thyroid Hormone Levels among Thai Pesticide Sprayers," *Toxics* 9, no. 1 (2021), doi.org/10.3390/toxics9010016.

5. Kheradpisheh, Z., M. Mirzaei, A. Mahvi, et al., "Impact of Drinking Water Fluoride on Human Thyroid Hormones: A Case-Control Study," *Scientific Reports* 8 (2018), doi.org/10.1038 /s41598-018-20696-4; and Dey, S. and B. Giri, "Fluoride Fact on Human Health and Health Problems: A Review." *Medical and Clinical Reviews* 2, no. 2 (2015), doi.org/10.21767/2471 -299x.1000011.

6. Goodman, C., M. Bashash, R. Green, et al., "Domain-specific Effects of Prenatal Fluoride Exposure on Child IQ at 4, 5, and 6–12 Years in the ELEMENT Cohort," *Environmental Research* 211, 112993 (2022), doi.org/10.1016/j.envres.2022.112993.

7. Ferreira, M., P. Nascimento, L. Bittencourt, et al., "Is There Any Association Between Fluoride Exposure and Thyroid Function Modulation? A Systematic Review," *PLOS One* 19 (2024), doi.org/10.1371/journal.pone.0301911.

8. Lisco, G., A. De Tullio, V. Giagulli, et al., "Interference on Iodine Uptake and Human Thyroid Function by Perchlorate-Contaminated Water and Food," *Nutrients* 12, no. 6 (2020), doi .org/10.3390/nu12061669; and Chac, D., D. Slater, Y. Guillaume, et al., "Association Between Chlorine-Treated Drinking Water, the Gut Microbiome, and Enteric Pathogen Burden in Young Children in Haiti: An Observational Study," *International Journal of Infectious Diseases* 147, 107165 (2024), doi.org/10.1016/j.ijid.2024.107165.

9. Qiu, Y., Y. Hu, Z. Xing, et al., "Birth Control Pills and Risk of Hypothyroidism: A Cross-Sectional Study of the National Health and Nutrition Examination Survey, 2007–2012," *BMJOpen* 11, no. 6 (2021), doi.org/10.1136/bmjopen-2020-046607.

10. Wiegratz, I., F. Kutschera, J. Lee, et al., "Effect of Four Different Oral Contraceptives on Various Sex Hormones and Serum-Binding Globulins," *Contraception* 67, no. 1 (2003): 25–32, doi .org/10.1016/s0010-7824(02)00436-5.

11. Torre, F., A. Calogero, R. Condorelli, et al., "Effects of Oral Contraceptives on Thyroid Function and Vice Versa," *Journal of Endocrinological Investigation* 43 (2020): 1181–88, doi.org /10.1007/s40618-020-01230-8.

12. Sabatino L., C. Vassalle, C. Del Seppia, et al., "Deiodinases and the Three Types of Thyroid Hormone Deiodination Reactions," *Endocrinology and Metabolism(Seoul)* 36, no. 5 (2021): 952–64, www.e-enm.org/journal/view.php?doi=10.3803/EnM.2021.1198.

13. Wiersinga, W., "Propranolol and Thyroid Hormone Metabolism," *Thyroid* 1, no. 3 (1991): 273–77, doi.org/10.1089/thy.1991.1.273.

14. Reiners, C., V. Drozd, and S. Yamashita, "Hypothyroidism after Radiation Exposure: Brief Narrative Review," *Journal of Neural Transmission* 127 (2020): 1455–66, www.link.springer .com/article/10.1007/s00702-020-02260-5.

Chapter 4: Thyropause or Menopause—or Both?

1. Nazneen, T., "Objective Evaluation of Thyroid Function in Postmenopausal Women," *National Journal of Physiology, Pharmacy and Pharmacology* 13, no. 8 (2023), doi.org/10.5455 /njppp.2023.13.01033202330012023.

2. He, Z., Q. Ouyang, Q. Chen, et al., "Molecular Mechanisms of Hypothalamic-Pituitary-Ovarian/Thyroid Axis Regulating Age at First Egg in Geese," *Poultry Science* 103, no. 3 (2024), doi.org/10.1016/j.psj.2024.103478.

3. Davison, S. L., R. Bell, S. Donath, et al., "Androgen Levels in Adult Females: Changes with Age, Menopause, and Oophorectomy," *Journal of Clinical Endocrinology and Metabolism* 90, no. 7 (2005): 3847–53, doi.org/10.1210/jc.2005-0212.

4. Ibid.

5. Torre, F., A. Calogero, R. Condorelli, et al., "Effects of Oral Contraceptives on Thyroid Function and Vice Versa," *Journal of Endocrinological Investigation* 43 (2020): 1181–88, doi.org /10.1007/s40618-020-01230-8; and Mazer, N., "Interaction of Estrogen Therapy and Thyroid Hormone Replacement in Postmenopausal Women," *Thyroid* 14, no. 1 (2004), doi.org /10.1089/105072504323024561.

6. Xie, J., J. Wang, and X. Cui, "Research Progress on Estrogen and Estrogen Receptors in the Occurrence and Progression of Autoimmune Thyroid Diseases," *Autoimmunity Reviews* 24, no. 6 (2025), doi.org/10.1016/j.autrev.2025.103803.

Chapter 5: What the Numbers *Really* Mean

1. Ken Berry and Kim Howerton, *Common Sense Labs: A Practical Guide to Decoding Your Blood Work and Taking Control of Your Health, Updated and Expanded Edition* (Las Vegas: Victory Belt Publishing, 2025).
2. Halsall, D. and S. Oddy, "Clinical and Laboratory Aspects of 3,3',5'-triiodothyronine (Reverse T3)," *Annals of Clinical Biochemistry: International Journal of Laboratory Medicine* 58, no. 1 (2020): 29–37, doi.org/10.1177/0004563220969150; and Chopra, I., U. Chopra, S. Smith, et al., "Reciprocal Changes in Serum Concentrations of 3,3',5'-Triiodothyronine (Reverse T3) and 3,3'5-Triiodothyronine (T3) in Systemic Illnesses," *Journal of Clinical Endocrinology and Metabolism* 41, no. 6 (1975): 1043–49, doi.org/10.1210/jcem-41-6-1043.
3. Kolanu, N., N. Awan, A. Butt, et al., "From Antibodies to Artificial Intelligence: A Comprehensive Review of Diagnostic Challenges in Hashimoto's Thyroiditis," *Cureus* 16, no. 2 (2024), doi.org/10.7759/cureus.54393.

Chapter 6: The Right Prescription

1. Wiersinga, W. M., "T4+T3 Combination Therapy: An Unsolved Problem of Increasing Magnitude and Complexity," *Endocrinology and Metabolism(Seoul)* 36, no. 5 (2021): 938–51, doi: 10.3803/EnM.2021.501.
2. Tsai, K., C. Long, T. Z. Liang, et al., "Driving Factors to Pursue Endocrinology Training Fellowship: Empirical Survey Data and Future Strategies," *Journal of Clinical Endocrinology and Metabolism* 107, no. 6 (2022), www.pubmed.ncbi.nlm.nih.gov/35165741/.
3. Penna, G. C., F. Salas-Lucia, M. O. Ribeiro, et al., "Gene Polymorphisms and Thyroid Hormone Signaling: Implication for the Treatment of Hypothyroidism," *Endocrine* 84, no. 2 (2024): 309–19, doi.org/10.1007/s12020-023-03528-y.

Chapter 8: Can I Heal My Thyroid Naturally?

1. Amin, B., and H. Hosseinzadeh, "Black Cumin (*Nigella sativa*) and Its Active Constituent, Thymoquinone: An Overview on the Analgesic and Anti-inflammatory Effects," *Planta Medica* 82 (2016): 8–16, doi.org/10.1055/s-0035-1557838.
2. Antonelli, A., P. Fallahi, S. Ferrari, et al., "3,5-diiodo-L-thyronine Increases Resting Metabolic Rate and Reduces Body Weight without Undesirable Side Effects," *Journal of Biological Regulators and Homeostatic Agents* 25, no. 4 (2011): 655–60, www.europepmc.org/article/med/22217997.
3. Ibid.
4. Kwon, H., K. Han, Y. Ku, et al., "The Effects of Resistance Training on Muscle and Body Fat Mass and Muscle Strength in Type 2 Diabetic Women," *Korean Diabetes Journal* 34, no. 2 (2010): 101–10, doi.org/10.4093/kdj.2010.34.2.101.
5. Schlienger, J., A. Anceau, G. Chabrier, et al., "Effect of Diabetic Control on the Level of Circulating Thyroid Hormones," *Diabetologia* 22 (1982): 486–88, doi.org/10.1007/bf00282596.

Chapter 9: Supplement Like You Mean It

1. Ghent, W., B. Eskin, D. Low, et al., "Iodine Replacement in Fibrocystic Disease of the Breast," *Canadian Journal of Surgery* 36, no. 5 (1993): 453–60, www.ncbi.nlm.nih.gov/pubmed/8221402.
2. Sorrenti, S., E. Baldini, D. Pironi, et al., "Iodine: Its Role in Thyroid Hormone Biosynthesis and Beyond," *Nutrients* 13, no. 12 (2021), doi.org/10.3390/nu13124469.

3. Roti, E. and E. Uberti, "Iodine Excess and Hyperthyroidism," *Thyroid* 11, no. 5 (2001): 493–500, doi.org/10.1089/105072501300176453.

4. Liu, S., X. Yu, Z. Xing, et al., "The Impact of Exposure to Iodine and Fluorine in Drinking Water on Thyroid Health and Intelligence in School-Age Children: A Cross-Sectional Investigation," *Nutrients* 16, no. 17 (2024), doi.org/10.3390/nu16172913; and Lisco, G., A. De Tullio, V. Giagulli, et al., "Interference on Iodine Uptake and Human Thyroid Function by Perchlorate-Contaminated Water and Food," *Nutrients* 12, no. 6 (2020), doi.org/10.3390/nu12061669.

5. Iamandii, I., L. De Pasquale, M. Giannone, et al., "Does Fluoride Exposure Affect Thyroid Function? A Systematic Review and Dose-Response Meta-Analysis," *Environmental Research* 242 (2023): 117759, doi.org/10.1016/j.envres.2023.117759.

6. Hall, M., R. Hornung, J. Chevrier, et al., "Fluoride Exposure and Thyroid Hormone Levels in Pregnancy: The MIREC Cohort," *Environment International* 184 (2024): 108442, doi.org/10.1016/j.envint.2024.108442.

7. Peckham, S., D. Lowery, and S. Spencer, "Are Fluoride Levels in Drinking Water Associated with Hypothyroidism Prevalence in England? A Large Observational Study of GP Practice Data and Fluoride Levels in Drinking Water," *Journal of Epidemiology & Community Health* 69, no. 7 (2015): 619–24, doi.org/10.1136/jech-2014-204971.

8. Larsen, P., and A. Zavacki, "Role of the Iodothyronine Deiodinases in the Physiology and Pathophysiology of Thyroid Hormone Action," *European Thyroid Journal* 1, no. 4 (2012): 232–42, doi.org/10.1159/000343922.

9. True Hope Nutritional Support, "What Is Nascent Iodine? And Why Is It Better for Your Thyroid?" Truehope.com, October 2, 2025, www.truehope.com/what-is-nascent-iodine-and-why-is-it-better-for-your-thyroid/.

10. www.betterlifedoctor.com, https://betterlifedoctor.com /products /iodine-fixxr?srsltid =AfmBOoqdY8jRXKFwV6L6GhP0lVs6VAhqtEJCtacUcHIkJ1c086o_iJwM.

11. Jeronimo F. Torti and Ricardo Correa, *Potassium Iodide* (Treasure Island, FL: StatPearls Publishing, 2025), www.ncbi.nlm.nih.gov/books/NBK542320/.

12. Wang, K., H. Wei, W. Zhang, et al., "Severely Low Serum Magnesium Is Associated with Increased Risks of Positive Anti-Thyroglobulin Antibody and Hypothyroidism: A Cross-Sectional Study," *Scientific Reports* 8, no. 1 (2018), www.pubmed.ncbi.nlm.nih.gov/29967483/.

13. Kolanu, B., S. Vadakedath, V. Boddula, et al., "Activities of Serum Magnesium and Thyroid Hormones in Pre-, Peri-, and Post-menopausal Women," *Cureus* 12, no. 1 (2020), doi.org/10.7759/cureus.6554.

14. Pickering, G., A. Mazur, M. Trousselard, et al., "Magnesium Status and Stress: The Vicious Circle Concept Revisited," *Nutrients* 12, no. 12 (2020), doi.org/10.3390/nu12123672.

15. Jones, J., P. Desper, S. Shane, et al., "Magnesium Metabolism in Hyperthyroidism and Hypothyroidism," *Journal of Clinical Investigation* 45, no. 6 (1966): 891–900, doi.org/10.1172/jci 105404.

16. Rondanelli, M., M. Faliva, A. Tartara, et al., "An Update on Magnesium and Bone Health," *BioMetals* 34 (2021): 715–36, doi.org/10.1007/s10534-021-00305-0.

17. Gobind, A., "The Role of Magnesium Supplement in Laryngopharyngeal Reflux Disease," *International Journal of Otorhinolaryngology and Head and Neck Surgery* 8, no. 1 (2021), doi.org/10.18203/issn.2454-5929.ijohns20214899.

18. Morishita, D., T. Tomita, S. Mori, et al., "Senna Versus Magnesium Oxide for the Treatment of Chronic Constipation: A Randomized, Placebo-Controlled Trial," *American Journal of Gastroenterology* 116, no. 1 (2020): 152–61, doi.org/10.14309/ajg.0000000000000942.

19. Zhang, Y., P. Xun, R. Wang, et al., "Can Magnesium Enhance Exercise Performance?" *Nutrients* 9, no. 9 (2017), doi.org/10.3390/nu9090946.

20. Hanna, M., E. Jaqua, V. Nguyen, et al., "B Vitamins: Functions and Uses in Medicine," *Permanente Journal* 26, no. 2 (2022): 89–97, doi.org/10.7812/tpp/21.204.

21. Doscherholmen, A., and W. Swaim, "Impaired Assimilation of Egg Co 57 Vitamin B$_{12}$ in Patients with Hypochlorhydria and Achlorhydria and after Gastric Resection," *Gastroenter-*

ology 64, no. 5 (1973): 913–19, doi.org/10.1016/s0016-5085(73)80002-2; and Cellini, M., M. Santaguida, C. Virili, et al., "Hashimoto's Thyroiditis and Autoimmune Gastritis," *Frontiers in Endocrinology* 8 (2017), doi.org/10.3389/fendo.2017.00092.

22. Dekker, M., G. Heerdink, and C. Plattel, "Vitamin B_{12} Deficiency-Induced Neuropathy and Cognitive and Motor Impairment in the Elderly: A Case Study," *Food and Nutrition Bulletin* 45 (2024): S53–S57, doi.org/10.1177/03795721241226886.

23. Krishnamurthy, H., S. Reddy, V. Jayaraman, et al., "Effect of Micronutrients on Thyroid Parameters," *Journal of Thyroid Research* (2021), doi.org/10.1155/2021/1865483.

24. Russo, S., F. Salas-Lucia, and A. Bianco, "Deiodinases and the Metabolic Code for Thyroid Hormone Action," *Endocrinology* 162, no. 8 (2021), doi.org/10.1210/endocr/bqab059.

25. Luo, D., B. Li, Z. Shan, et al., "The Impacts of Vitamin D Supplementation on Serum Levels of Thyroid Autoantibodies in Patients with Autoimmune Thyroid Disease: A Meta-Analysis," *PeerJ* 13 (2025), doi.org/10.7717/peerj.19541; and Leko, M., I. Jureško, L. Rozić, et al., "Vitamin D and the Thyroid: A Critical Review of the Current Evidence," *International Journal of Molecular Sciences* 24, no. 4 (2023), doi.org/10.3390/ijms24043586.

26. Sassi, F., C. Tamone, and P. D'Amelio, "Vitamin D: Nutrient, Hormone, and Immunomodulator," *Nutrients* 10, no. 11 (2018), doi.org/10.3390/nu10111656.

27. Yang, L., P. Yun, and F. Li, "Association between Vitamin D Serum Levels and Thyroid Cancer: A Meta-Analysis," *Frontiers in Endocrinology* 16 (2025), doi.org/10.3389/fendo.2025 .1602844.

28. Lundqvist, J., "Vitamin D as a Regulator of Steroidogenic Enzymes," *F1000Research*, 3 (2014): 155, doi.org/10.12688/f1000research.4714.1.

29. Theofilus, G., B. Wisnu, W. Desy, et al., "Effect Nigella Sativa Extract for Balancing Immune Response in Pristane Induced Lupus Mice Model," *Journal of Applied Pharmaceutical Science* 11, no. 7 (2020), doi.org/10.7324/japs.2021.110716.

30. Kavyani, Z., V. Musazadeh, S. Golpour-Hamedani, et al., "The Effect of Nigella sativa (Black Seed) on Biomarkers of Inflammation and Oxidative Stress: An Updated Systematic Review and Meta-analysis of Randomized Controlled Trials," *Inflammopharmacology* 31 (2023): 1149–65, doi.org/10.1007/s10787-023-01213-0.

31. Osowiecka, K., and J. Myszkowska-Ryciak, "The Influence of Nutritional Intervention in the Treatment of Hashimoto's Thyroiditis—A Systematic Review," *Nutrients* 15, no. 4 (2023), doi .org/10.3390/nu15041041.

32. Farhangi, M., and S. Tajmiri, "The Effects of Powdered Black Cumin Seeds on Markers of Oxidative Stress, Intracellular Adhesion Molecule (ICAM)-1 and Vascular Cell Adhesion Molecule (VCAM)-1 in Patients with Hashimoto's Thyroiditis," *Clinical Nutrition ESPEN* 37 (2020): 207–12, doi.org/10.1016/j.clnesp.2020.02.015.

33. Tajmiri, S., M. Farhangi, and P. Dehghan, "Nigella Sativa Treatment and Serum Concentrations of Thyroid Hormones, Transforming Growth Factor ß (TGF-ß) and Interleukin 23 (IL-23) in Patients with Hashimoto's Thyroiditis," *European Journal of Integrative Medicine* 8, no. 4 (2016): 576–80, doi.org/10.1016/j.eujim.2016.03.003.

34. Abdelwahab, M., E. Mohamed, and E. Fahmy, "Effect of Low Caloric Diet Supplemented by Fennel (Foeniculum vulgare) Seeds or Black Cumin (Nigella sativa) Seeds and Its Mixture on Obese Adult Female Patients," *African Journal of Biological Sciences* 17, no. 1 (2021), doi.org /10.21608/ajbs.2021.191214; and Maideen, N., "Nigella Sativa (Black seeds)—Potential Herb to Help Weight Loss," *Current Traditional Medicine* 8, no. 4 (2021), https://doi.org/10.2174 /2215083807666211109115834.

35. Bashir, K., J. Kim, J. Kim, et al., "Efficacy Confirmation Test of Black Cumin (Nigella sativa L.) Seeds Extract Using a High-Fat Diet Mouse Model," *Metabolites* 13, no. 4 (2023), doi.org /10.3390/metabo13040501.

36. Zielińska, M., K. Dereń, E. Polak-Szczybyło, et al., "The Role of Bioactive Compounds of Nigella sativa in Rheumatoid Arthritis Therapy—Current Reports," *Nutrients* 13, no. 10 (2021), doi.org/10.3390/nu13103369; and Nazakat, L., S. Ali, M. Summer, et al., "Pharmacological

Modes of Plant-Derived Compounds for Targeting Inflammation in Rheumatoid Arthritis: A Comprehensive Review on Immunomodulatory Perspective," *Inflammopharmacology* 33 (2025): 1537–81, doi.org/10.1007/s10787-025-01664-7.

37. Saadat, S., M. Aslani, V. Ghorani, et al., "The Effects of Nigella sativa on Respiratory, Allergic and Immunologic Disorders, Evidence from Experimental and Clinical Studies, A Comprehensive and Updated Review," *Phytotherapy Research* 35, no. 6 (2021): 2968–96, doi.org/10.1002/ptr.7003.

38. Hajhashemi, V., A. Ghannadi, and H. Jafarabadi, "Black Cumin Seed Essential Oil, as a Potent Analgesic and Antiinflammatory Drug," *Phytotherapy Research* 18, no. 3 (2024): 195–99, doi.org/10.1002/ptr.1390.

39. Rounagh, M., V. Musazadeh, A. Hosseininejad-Mohebati, et al., "Effects of Nigella sativa Supplementation on Lipid Profiles in Adults: An Updated Systematic Review and Meta-analysis of Randomized Controlled Trials," *Clinical Nutrition ESPEN* 61 (2024): 168–80, doi.org/10.1016/j.clnesp.2024.03.020.

40. Kavyani, Z., V. Musazadeh, E. Safaei, et al., "Antihypertensive Effects of Nigella sativa Supplementation: An Updated Systematic Review and Meta-analysis of Randomized Controlled Trials," *Phytotherapy Research* 37, no. 8 (2023): 3224–38, doi.org/10.1002/ptr.7891.

41. Shafiq, H., A. Ahmad, T. Masud, et al., "Cardio-protective and Anti-cancer Therapeutic Potential of Nigella sativa," *Iranian Journal of Basic Medical Sciences* 17, no. 12 (2014): 967–79, www.ijbms.mums.ac.ir/article_3853.html.

42. Majdalawieh, A., M. Fayyad, and G. Nasrallah, "Anti-cancer Properties and Mechanisms of Action of Thymoquinone, the Major Active Ingredient of Nigella sativa," *Critical Reviews in Food Science and Nutrition* 57, no. 18 (2017): 3911–28, doi.org/10.1080/10408398.2016.1277971; and Sourav, C., K. Chong, and H. Tayara, "Exploring Nigella sativa Anticancer Properties Using Network Pharmacology and Molecular Docking Approach for Non-Small Cell Lung Cancer," *Food Bioscience* 63 (2025), doi.org/10.1016/j.fbio.2024.105525.

43. Schomburg, L., and J. Köhrle, "On the Importance of Selenium and Iodine Metabolism for Thyroid Hormone Biosynthesis and Human Health," *Molecular Nutrition & Food Research* 52, no. 11 (2008): 1235–46, doi.org/10.1002/mnfr.200700465.

44. Wang, F., C. Li, S. Li, et al., "Selenium and Thyroid Diseases," *Frontiers in Endocrinology* 14 (2023), doi.org /10.3389 /fendo.2023.1133000.

45. Gärtner, R., B. Gasnier, J. Dietrich, et al., "Selenium Supplementation in Patients with Autoimmune Thyroiditis Decreases Thyroid Peroxidase Antibodies Concentrations," *Journal of Clinical Endocrinology and Metabolism* 87, no. 4 (2002): 1687–91, doi.org/10.1210/jcem.87.4.8421.

46. Haddad, S., and M. Houssaini, "Effects of Ashwagandha Supplements on Cortisol, Stress, and Anxiety Levels in Adults: A Systematic Review and Meta-Analysis," *British Journal of Psychiatry Open* 11 (2025): S39–S39, doi.org/10.1192/bjo.2025.10136.

47. Xie, W., F. Su, G. Wang, et al., "Glucose-lowering Effect of Berberine on Type 2 Diabetes: A Systematic Review and Meta-analysis," *Frontiers in Pharmacology* 13 (2022), doi.org/10.3389/fphar.2022.1015045; and Zhao, J., X. Huang, J. Zhang, et al., "Overall and Sex-Specific Effect of Berberine on Glycemic and Insulin-Related Traits: A Systematic Review and Meta-analysis of Randomized Controlled Trials," *Journal of Nutrition* 153, no. 10 (2023): 2939–50, doi.org/10.1016/j.tjnut.2023.08.016.

48. Henkel, R., R. Wang, S. Bassett, et al., "Tongkat Ali as a Potential Herbal Supplement for Physically Active Male and Female Seniors—A Pilot Study," *Phytotherapy Research* 28, no. 4 (2014): 544–50, doi.org/10.1002/ptr.5017; and Talbott, S., J. Talbott, A. George, et al., "Effect of Tongkat Ali on Stress Hormones and Psychological Mood State in Moderately Stressed Subjects," *Journal of the International Society of Sports Nutrition* 10, no. 1 (2013), doi.org/10.1186/1550-2783-10-28.

49. Alomari, T., H. Al-Abdallat, R. Hamamreh, et al., "Assessing the Antiviral Potential of Melatonin: A Comprehensive Systematic Review," *Reviews in Medical Virology* 34, no. 1 (2023), doi.org/10.1002/rmv.2499.

50. Ribeiro, F., S. Forbes, D. Candow, et al., "Creatine Supplementation and Muscle-Brain Axis: A New Possible Mechanism?" *Frontiers in Nutrition* 12 (2025), doi.org/10.3389/fnut.2025.15 79204.

51. Neelab, J., A. Zeb, and M. Jamil, "Milk Thistle Protects Against Non-alcoholic Fatty Liver Disease Induced by Dietary Thermally Oxidized Tallow," *Heliyon* 10, no. 10 (2024), doi.org/10.1016/j.heliyon.2024.e31445.

Chapter 10: T2

1. Antonelli, A., P. Fallahi, S. Ferrari, et al., "3,5-diiodo-L-thyronine Increases Resting Metabolic Rate and Reduces Body Weight without Undesirable Side Effects," *Journal of Biological Regulators and Homeostatic Agents* 25, no. 4 (2011): 655–60, www.europepmc.org/article/med/22217997.

2. Grasselli, E., A. Voci, I. Demori, et al., "3,5-Diiodo-L-thyronine Modulates the Expression of Genes of Lipid Metabolism in a Rat Model of Fatty Liver," *Journal of Endocrinology* 212, no. 2 (2012): 149–58, doi.org/10.1530/joe-11-0288; and Petito, G., F. Cioffi, E. Silvestri, et al., "3,5-Diiodo-L-Thyronine (T2) Administration Affects Visceral Adipose Tissue Inflammatory State in Rats Receiving Long-Lasting High-Fat Diet," *Frontiers in Endocrinology* 12 (2021), doi.org/10.3389/fendo.2021.703170.

3. Giammanco, M., C. Di Liegro, G. Schiera, et al., "Genomic and Non-Genomic Mechanisms of Action of Thyroid Hormones and Their Catabolite 3,5-Diiodo-L-Thyronine in Mammals," *International Journal of Molecular Sciences* 21, no. 11 (2020), doi.org/10.3390/ijms21114140.

4. Cioffi, F., R. Senese, G. Petito, et al., "Both 3,3',5-triiodothyronine and 3,5-diodo-L-thyronine Are Able to Repair Mitochondrial DNA Damage but by Different Mechanisms," *Frontiers in Endocrinology* 10 (2019), doi.org/10.3389/fendo.2019.00216.

5. Antonelli, Fallahi, Ferrari, et al., "3,5-diiodo-L-thyronine Increases Resting Metabolic Rate and Reduces Body Weight without Undesirable Side Effects."

6. Senese, R., F. Cioffi, R. De Matteis, et al., "3,5 Diiodo-l-Thyronine (T2) Promotes the Browning of White Adipose Tissue in High-Fat Diet-Induced Overweight Male Rats Housed at Thermoneutrality," *Cells* 8, no. 3 (2019), doi.org/10.3390/cells8030256.

7. Lombardi, A., R. Senese, R. De Matteis, et al., "3,5-Diiodo-L-Thyronine Activates Brown Adipose Tissue Thermogenesis in Hypothyroid Rats," *PLOS One* 10 (2015), doi.org/10.1371/journal.pone.0116498.

8. Petito, G., F. Cioffi, N. Magnacca, et al., "Adipose Tissue Remodeling in Obesity: An Overview of the Actions of Thyroid Hormones and Their Derivatives," *Pharmaceuticals* 16, no. 4 (2023), doi.org/10.3390/ph16040572.

9. Chen, T., H. Wang, C. Chang, et al., "Mitochondrial Glutathione in Cellular Redox Homeostasis and Disease Manifestation," *International Journal of Molecular Sciences* 25, no. 2 (2024), doi.org/10.3390/ijms25021314.

Chapter 11: Eat This, Not That

1. Akçay, M. N., and G. Akçay, "The Presence of the Antigliadin Antibodies in Autoimmune Thyroid Diseases," *Hepatogastroenterology* (2003), www.pubmed.ncbi.nlm.nih.gov/15244201.

2. Liikonen, V., C. Gomez-Gallego, and M. Kolehmainen, "The Effects of Whole Grain Cereals on Tryptophan Metabolism and Intestinal Barrier Function: Underlying Factors of Health Impact," *Proceedings of the Nutrition Society* 83, no. 1 (2024): 42–54, doi.org/10.1017/s0029665123003671.

3. Kazemi, A., J. Speakman, S. Soltani, et al., "Effect of Calorie Restriction or Protein Intake on Circulating Levels of Insulin Like Growth Factor I in Humans: A Systematic Review and Meta-analysis," *Clinical Nutrition* 39, no. 6 (2020): 1705–16, doi.org/10.1016/j.clnu.2019.07.030.

4. Maleky, F., and L. Ahmadi, "Adhering to Recommended Dietary Protein Intake for Optimizing Human Health Benefits Versus Exceeding Levels," *RSC Advances* 12 (2025): 9230–42, doi.org/10.1039/d4ra08221d.

5. Shevkani, Khetan, and Shivani Chourasia, "Dietary Proteins: Functions, Health Benefits and Healthy Aging" in *Nutrition, Food and Diet in Ageing and Longevity*, ed. Suresh I. S. Rattan and Gurcharan Kaur (Princeton, NJ: Springer Publishing, 2021), doi.org/10.1007/978-3-030-83 017-5_1.

6. Carbone, J., and S. Pasiakos, "Dietary Protein and Muscle Mass: Translating Science to Application and Health Benefit," *Nutrients* 11, no. 5 (2019), doi.org/10.3390/nu11051136.

7. Stokes, T., A. Hector, R. Morton, et al., "Recent Perspectives Regarding the Role of Dietary Protein for the Promotion of Muscle Hypertrophy with Resistance Exercise Training," *Nutrients* 10, no. 2 (2018), doi.org/10.3390/nu10020180.

8. Latoch, A., D. Stasiak, and P. Siczek, "Edible Offal as a Valuable Source of Nutrients in the Diet—A Review," *Nutrients* 16, no. 11 (2024), doi.org/10.3390/nu16111609.

9. Wan, S., X. Zhou, F. Xie, et al., "Ketogenic Diet and Cancer: Multidimensional Exploration and Research," *Science China Life Sciences* 68 (2025): 1010–24, doi.org/10.1007/s11427 -023-2637-2; and Halma, M., J. Tuszynski, and P. Marik, "Cancer Metabolism as a Therapeutic Target and Review of Interventions." *Nutrients* 15, no. 19 (2023), doi.org/10.3390/nu15 194245.

10. Iacovides, S., S. Maloney, S. Bhana, et al., "Could the Ketogenic Diet Induce a Shift in Thyroid Function and Support a Metabolic Advantage in Healthy Participants? A Pilot Randomized-Controlled-Crossover Trial," *PLOS One* 17 (2022), doi.org/10.1371 /journal.pone.0269440.

11. Laffond, A., C. Rivera-Picón, P. Rodríguez-Muñoz, et al., "Mediterranean Diet for Primary and Secondary Prevention of Cardiovascular Disease and Mortality: An Updated Systematic Review," *Nutrients* 15, no. 15 (2023), doi.org/10.3390/nu15153356.

Chapter 12: Lift Heavy Sh*t

1. Thyfault, J., and A. Bergouignan, "Exercise and Metabolic Health: Beyond Skeletal Muscle," *Diabetologia* 63 (2020): 1464–74, doi.org/10.1007/s00125-020-05177-6; and Momma, H., R. Kawakami, T. Honda, et al., "Muscle-strengthening Activities Are Associated with Lower Risk and Mortality in Major Non-Communicable Diseases: A Systematic Review and Meta-Analysis of Cohort Studies," *British Journal of Sports Medicine* 56, no. 13 (2022): 755–63, doi.org/10.1136/bjsports-2021-105061.

2. Bernárdez-Vázquez, R., J. Raya-González, D. Castillo, et al., "Resistance Training Variables for Optimization of Muscle Hypertrophy: An Umbrella Review," *Frontiers in Sports and Active Living* 4 (2022), doi.org/10.3389/fspor.2022.949021.

3. Zhao, F., W. Su, Y. Sun, et al., "Optimal Resistance Training Parameters for Improving Bone Mineral Density in Postmenopausal Women: A Systematic Review and Meta-Analysis," *Journal of Orthopaedic Surgery and Research* 20 (2025), doi.org/10.1186/s13018-025-05890-1.

4. Nazir, A., H. Heryaman, C. Juli, et al., "Resistance Training in Cardiovascular Diseases: A Review on Its Effectiveness in Controlling Risk Factors," *Integrated Blood Pressure Control* 17 (2024): 21–37, doi.org/10.2147/ibpc.s449086.

5. Zurlo, F., K. Larson, C. Bogardus, et al., "Skeletal Muscle Metabolism Is a Major Determinant of Resting Energy Expenditure," *Journal of Clinical Investigation* 86, no. 5 (1990): 1423–27, doi.org/10.1172/jci114857.

Chapter 13: Lower Your Toxic Load

1. Plunk, E., and S. Richards, "Endocrine-Disrupting Air Pollutants and Their Effects on the Hypothalamus-Pituitary-Gonadal Axis," *International Journal of Molecular Sciences* 21, no. 23 (2020), doi.org/10.3390/ijms21239191.

2. Vobecky, M., and A. Babický, "Effect of Enhanced Bromide Intake on the Concentration Ratio I/Br in the Rat Thyroid Gland," *Biological Trace Element Research* 43 (2008): 509–16, doi.org/10.1007/bf02917354.

3. Rafi'i, M., M. Ja'afar, M. Nawi, et al., "Association between Toxic Heavy Metals and Non-cancerous Thyroid Disease: A Scoping Review," *PeerJ* 13 (2025), doi.org/10.7717/peerj.18962.

4. Kim, K., M. Argos, V. Persky, et al., "Associations of Exposure to Metal and Metal Mixtures with Thyroid Hormones: Results from the NHANES 2007–2012," *Environmental Research* 212, part C (2022), doi.org/10.1016/j.envres.2022.113413.

5. De Lima, N., J. Camilo, P. Carmo, et al., "Subacute Exposure to Lead Promotes Disruption in the Thyroid Gland Function in Male and Female Rats," *Environmental Pollution* 274 (2020), doi.org/10.1016/j.envpol.2020.115889.

6. Buha, A., V. Matović, B. Antonijević, et al., "Overview of Cadmium Thyroid Disrupting Effects and Mechanisms," *International Journal of Molecular Sciences* 19, no. 5 (2018), doi.org/10.3390/ijms19051501.

7. Esform, A., T. Farkhondeh, S. Samarghandian, et al., "Environmental Arsenic Exposure and Its Toxicological Effect on Thyroid Function: A Systematic Review," *Reviews on Environmental Health* 37, no. 2 (2022): 281–89, doi.org/10.1515/reveh-2021-0025.

8. Moriyama, K., T. Tagami, T. Akamizu, et al., "Thyroid Hormone Action Is Disrupted by Bisphenol A as an Antagonist," *Journal of Clinical Endocrinology and Metabolism* 87, no. 11 (2002): 5185–90, doi.org/10.1210/jc.2002-020209.

9. Gorini F., E. Bustaffa, A. Coi, et al., "Bisphenols as Environmental Triggers of Thyroid Dysfunction: Clues and Evidence," *International Journal of Environmental Research and Public Health* 17, no. 8 (2020), doi.org/10.3390/ijerph17082654.

10. Leonard J. A., Y. M. Tan, M. Gilbert, et al., "Estimating Margin of Exposure to Thyroid Peroxidase Inhibitors Using High-Throughput In Vitro Data, High-Throughput Exposure Modeling, and Physiologically Based Pharmacokinetic/Pharmacodynamic Modeling," *Toxicological Sciences* 151, no. 1 (2016): 57–70, doi:10.1093/toxsci/kfw022.

11. Hernández, A., S. Bennekou, A. Hart, et al., "Mechanisms Underlying Disruptive Effects of Pesticides on the Thyroid Function," *Current Opinion in Toxicology* 19 (2020): 34–41, doi.org/10.1016/j.cotox.2019.10.003.

12. Ibid.

13. Lima, C., M. Falcão, J. Rosa, et al., "Pesticides and Their Impairing Effects on Epithelial Barrier Integrity, Dysbiosis, Disruption of the AhR Signaling Pathway and Development of Immune-Mediated Inflammatory Diseases," *International Journal of Molecular Sciences* 23, no. 20 (2022), doi.org/10.3390/ijms232012402.

14. Liu, C., L. Zhao, L. Wei, et al., "DEHP Reduces Thyroid Hormones via Interacting with Hormone Synthesis-Related Proteins, Deiodinases, Transthyretin, Receptors, and Hepatic Enzymes in Rats," *Environmental Science and Pollution Research* 22 (2015): 12711–19, doi.org/10.1007/s11356-015-4567-7.

15. Yan, M., H. Zhu, H. Luo, et al., "Daily Exposure to Environmental Volatile Organic Compounds Triggers Oxidative Damage: Evidence from a Large-Scale Survey in China," *Environmental Science & Technology* 57, no. 49 (2023), doi.org/10.1021/acs.est.3c06055.

16. Zhang, M., J. Shi, B. Li, et al., "Thyroid Hormone Receptor Agonistic and Antagonistic Activity of Newly Synthesized Dihydroxylated Polybrominated Diphenyl Ethers: An In Vitro and In Silico Coactivator Recruitment Study," *Toxics* 12, no. 4 (2024), doi.org/10.3390/toxics12040281.

17. Oulhote, Y., J. Chevrier, and M. F. Bouchard, "Exposure to Polybrominated Diphenyl Ethers (PBDEs) and Hypothyroidism in Canadian Women," *Journal of Clinical Endocrinology & Metabolism* 101, no. 2 (2016): 590–98, doi.org/10.1210/jc.2015-2659; and Allen, J. G., S. Gale, R. T. Zoeller, et al., "PBDE Flame Retardants, Thyroid Disease, and Menopausal Status in U.S. Women," *Environmental Health* 15, no. 1 (2016), doi.org/10.1186/s12940-016-0141-0.

Chapter 14: Flip Stress on Its Head

1. Bianco, A., M. Nunes, N. Hell, et al., "The Role of Glucocorticoids in the Stress Induced Reduction of Extrathyroidal 3,5,3'-Triiodothyronine Generation in Rats," *Endocrinology* 120, no. 3 (1987): 1033–38, doi.org/10.1210/endo-120-3-1033.
2. Javid, M., S. U. Khan, M. Akram, et al. "Higher Cortisol Level and Reduced Circulating Triiodothyronine in Patients with Cardiovascular Diseases: A Case-Control Study," *JRSM Cardiovasc Disease* 14 (2025), doi.org/10.1177/20480040251340609.
3. Liao, L., Y. He, L. Li, et al., "A Preliminary Review of Studies on Adaptogens: Comparison of Their Bioactivity in TCM with that of Ginseng-Like Herbs Used Worldwide," *Chinese Medicine* 13, no. 57 (2018), doi.org/10.1186/s13020-018-0214-9.
4. Kim, H., B. Huang, and A. Spector, "Phosphatidylserine in the Brain: Metabolism and Function," *Progress in Lipid Research* 56 (2014): 1–18, doi.org/10.1016/j.plipres.2014.06.002.
5. Ibid.
6. Cohen, M., "Tulsi-Ocimum sanctum: An Herb for All Reasons," *Journal of Ayurveda and Integrative Medicine* 5, no. 4 (2014): 251–59, www.pmc.ncbi.nlm.nih.gov/articles/PMC 4296439.
7. Xia, N., J. Li, H. Wang, et al., "Schisandra chinensis and Rhodiola rosea Exert an Anti-Stress Effect on the HPA Axis and Reduce Hypothalamic C-Fos Expression in Rats Subjected to Repeated Stress," *Experimental and Therapeutic Medicine* 11, no. 1 (2016): 353–59, doi.org/10.3892/etm.2015.2882.
8. Das, G., H. Shin, G. Leyva-Gómez, et al., "Cordyceps spp.: A Review on Its Immune-Stimulatory and Other Biological Potentials," *Frontiers in Pharmacology* 11 (2021), doi.org/10.3389/fphar.2020.602364.
9. Yao, C., Z. Wang, H. Jiang, et al., "Ganoderma lucidum Promotes Sleep Through a Gut Microbiota-Dependent and Serotonin-Involved Pathway in Mice," *Scientific Reports* 11 (2021), doi.org/10.1038/s41598-021-92913-6.
10. Adineh, H., M. Naderi, M. Yousefi, et al., "Dietary licorice (Glycyrrhiza glabra) Improves Growth, Lipid Metabolism, Antioxidant and Immune Responses, and Resistance to Crowding Stress in Common Carp, Cyprinus carpio," *Aquaculture Nutrition* (2020), doi.org/10.1111/anu.13194.

Chapter 15: Biohacking Breakthroughs

1. Kopp, K., E. Glotfelty, Y. Li, et al., "Glucagon-like Peptide-1 (GLP-1) Receptor Agonists and Neuroinflammation: Implications for Neurodegenerative Disease Treatment," *Pharmacological Research* 186 (2022), doi.org/10.1016/j.phrs.2022.106550.
2. Ussher, J., and D. Drucker, "Glucagon-like Peptide 1 Receptor Agonists: Cardiovascular Benefits and Mechanisms of Action," *Nature Reviews Cardiology* 20 (2023): 463–74, doi.org/10.1038/s41569-023-00849-3.
3. Liao, C., X. Liang, X. Zhang, et al., "The Effects of GLP-1 Receptor Agonists on Visceral Fat and Liver Ectopic Fat in an Adult Population with or without Diabetes and Nonalcoholic Fatty Liver Disease: A Systematic Review and Meta-Analysis," *PLOS One* 18 (2023), doi.org/10.1371/journal.pone.0289616; and Mantovani, A., G. Petracca, G. Beatrice, et al., "Glucagon-Like Peptide-1 Receptor Agonists for Treatment of Nonalcoholic Fatty Liver Disease and Nonalcoholic Steatohepatitis: An Updated Meta-Analysis of Randomized Controlled Trials," *Metabolites* 11, no. 2 (2021), doi.org/10.3390/metabo11020073.
4. Kopp, Glotfelty, Li, et al., "Glucagon-like Peptide-1 (GLP-1) Receptor Agonists and Neuroinflammation: Implications for Neurodegenerative Disease Treatment"; and Halloum, W., Y. Dughem, D. Beier, et al., "Glucagon-like Peptide-1 (GLP-1) Receptor Agonists for Headache and Pain Disorders: A Systematic Review," *Journal of Headache and Pain* 25 (2024), doi.org/10.1186/s10194-024-01821-3.
5. Berisha-Muharremi, V., B. Tahirbegolli, R. Phypers, et al., "Efficacy of Combined Photobiomodulation Therapy with Supplements versus Supplements alone in Restoring Thyroid Gland

Homeostasis in Hashimoto Thyroiditis: A Clinical Feasibility Parallel Trial with 6-Months Follow-Up," *Journal of Personalized Medicine* 13, no. 8 (2023), doi.org/10.3390/jpm13081274.

6. Hamblin, M., "Mechanisms and Applications of the Anti-inflammatory Effects of Photobiomodulation," *AIMS Biophysics* 4 (2017): 337–61, doi.org/10.3934/biophy.2017.3.337.

7. Ibid.

8. Adıgüzel, Ş., D. Akyurt, G. Özgen, et al., "The Effect of Cold Application to the Lateral Neck Area on Peripheral Vascular Access Pain: A Randomised Controlled Study," *Journal of Clinical Medicine* 12, no. 19 (2023), doi.org/10.3390/jcm12196273.

9. Torretta, E., M. Moriggi, D. Capitanio, et al., "Effects of Pulsed Electromagnetic Field Treatment on Skeletal Muscle Tissue Recovery in a Rat Model of Collagenase-Induced Tendinopathy: Results from a Proteome Analysis," *International Journal of Molecular Sciences* 25, no. 16 (2024), doi.org/10.3390/ijms25168852.

10. Chevalier, G., S. Sinatra, J. Oschman, et al., "Earthing: Health Implications of Reconnecting the Human Body to the Earth's Surface Electrons," *Journal of Environmental and Public Health* (2012), doi.org/10.1155/2012/291541.

Index

About the Author

Dr. Amie Hornaman, also known as "The Thyroid Fixer," is the CEO and founder of the Advanced Thyroid and Hormone Clinic, an international telehealth practice serving patients across the US and Canada. She also hosts the top-rated podcast *The Thyroid Fixer*, where she empowers listeners with the truth about thyroid health, hormones, and functional medicine. A sought-after speaker and author, Dr. Amie has been featured in documentaries including *sHEALed* (Amazon Prime), *Ageless*, and *Hormones, Health, and Harmony*. She is a trusted expert for *Forbes Health*, *Women's World*, *Daily Mail*, CBS News, Fox News, and Poosh.

Dr. Amie is also the creator of the Fixxr® Formula supplements, a science-backed nutraceutical line designed to support metabolism, energy, libido, and hormone balance. Driven by her own experience with thyroid and hormone misdiagnoses, Dr. Amie blends empathy with functional medicine to deliver lasting results. Her mission: optimize health, restore life, and help every patient step fully into the badass human they were meant to be.